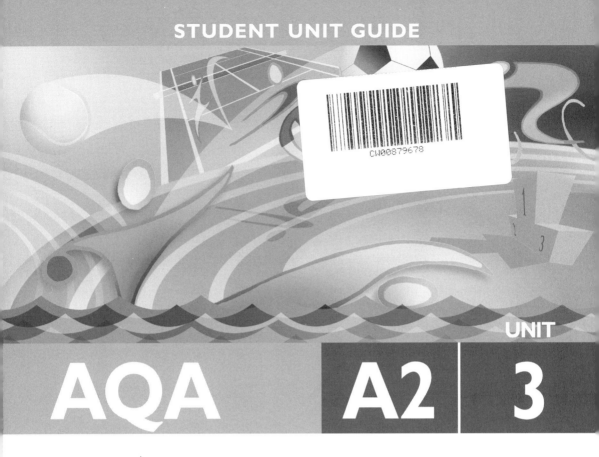

CW00879678

UNIT

AQA | A2 | 3

Physical Education

Optimising Performance and Evaluating Contemporary Issues within Sport

Symond Burrows, Michaela Byrne and Sue Young

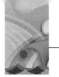
Philip Allan Updates, an imprint of Hodder Education, an Hachette UK company, Market Place, Deddington, Oxfordshire OX15 0SE

Orders
Bookpoint Ltd, 130 Milton Park, Abingdon, Oxfordshire OX14 4SB
tel: 01235 827720
fax: 01235 400454
e-mail: uk.orders@bookpoint.co.uk
Lines are open 9.00 a.m.–5.00 p.m., Monday to Saturday, with a 24-hour message answering service. You can also order through the Philip Allan Updates website: www.philipallan.co.uk

© Philip Allan Updates 2010

ISBN 978-0-340-94786-9

First printed 2010
Impression number 5 4 3 2
Year 2014 2013 2012 2011 2010

All rights reserved; no part of this publication may be reproduced, stored in a retrieval system, or transmitted, in any other form or by any means, electronic, mechanical, photocopying, recording or otherwise without either the prior written permission of Philip Allan Updates or a licence permitting restricted copying in the United Kingdom issued by the Copyright Licensing Agency Ltd, Saffron House, 6–10 Kirby Street, London EC1N 8TS.

This guide has been written specifically to support students preparing for the AQA A2 Physical Education Unit 3 examination. The content has been neither approved nor endorsed by AQA and remains the sole responsibility of the author.

Typeset by Philip Allan Updates

Printed by MPG Books, Bodmin

Hachette UK's policy is to use papers that are natural, renewable and recyclable products and made from wood grown in sustainable forests. The logging and manufacturing processes are expected to conform to the environmental regulations of the country of origin.

P01607

Contents

Introduction

About this guide... 5

The specification.. 5

Study skills and revision strategies.. 6

The Unit 3 exam.. 8

■ ■ ■

Content Guidance

About this section 10

Applied physiology to optimise performance

Energy sources and systems 11

Causes of fatigue and the recovery process 15

What makes a successful endurance performance? 18

Structure and function of muscles.. 21

Sports supplements and ergogenic aids 25

Specialised training 28

Sports injuries... 31

Mechanics of movement.. 32

Psychological aspects that optimise performance

Personality.. 38

Arousal... 42

Controlling anxiety 47

Attitudes... 52

Aggression 55

Confidence 58

Attribution theory 62

Group success 64

Leadership 68

Evaluating contemporary influences in sport

Concepts and characteristics of World Games.. 71

The 'Olympic ideal' and its place in modern-day sport 76

Sport, deviance and the law.. 82

Commercialisation in modern-day sport.. 86

■ ■ ■

Questions and Answers

About this section 92

Q1 Energy sources and systems 93

Q2 Causes of fatigue and the recovery process 94

Q3 What makes a successful endurance performance? 96

Q4 Structure and function of muscles 97

Q5 Sports supplements and ergogenic aids 97

Q6 Specialised training 98

Q7 Sports injuries 99

Q8 Mechanics of movement 100

Q9 Arousal 101

Q10 Confidence 102

Q11 Attribution theory 103

Q12 Leadership 104

Q13 Concepts and characteristics of World Games 105

Q14 The 'Olympic ideal' and its place in sport today 107

Q15 Sport, deviance and the law 108

Q16 Commercialisation in modern-day sport 109

Introduction
About this guide

This unit guide is written to help you prepare for the AQA PE Unit 3 exam. The exam covers the A2 theoretical content of three separate aspects of PE:

- applied physiology to optimise performance
- psychological aspects that optimise performance
- evaluating contemporary issues and their influence on the performer

This **Introduction** provides advice on how to use the unit guide and some suggestions for effective revision. Each aspect of the specification required for the Unit 3 test is covered in the **Content Guidance**. The **Questions and Answers** section provides examples of questions from various topic areas, together with student answers and examiner comments on how these could have been improved.

The specification

Unit 3 is about the optimisation of performance. The specification describes the aspects of PE that you need to learn. If you do not have a copy of the specification, ask your teacher or download it from the AQA website (**www.aqa.org.uk**).

The examiners will pay careful attention to the specification when setting questions for the A-level exam. If it is not in the specification, it will not be examined. If it is in the specification, it *could* be examined.

In addition to describing the content of the course (which sometimes provides detail that could earn you marks), the specification gives information about the unit tests and about other skills required — for example, using the experience gained by performing practical activities as a basis for improving physiological and psychological understanding. You also need to develop the skills of interpreting and drawing graphs and diagrams.

You might find it useful to read the examiners' reports and mark schemes from previous unit tests (available from AQA). These demonstrate the depth of knowledge examiners are looking for, as well as pointing out common mistakes and providing advice on how to achieve good grades.

Study skills and revision strategies

Effective study skills and revision strategies are an important part of ensuring success in your A-level PE exam. This section of the guide provides advice on how to study this subject, together with some strategies you should consider adopting to ensure your revision is effective.

Organising your notes

As an A-level PE student you will accumulate a lot of notes. It is important to keep this information in an organised manner. Good notes should be clear and concise. You could try to organise them under main headings and subheadings, with key points highlighted using capitals or colours. Numbered lists can be useful, as can the presentation of information in table form and simple diagrams. For example:

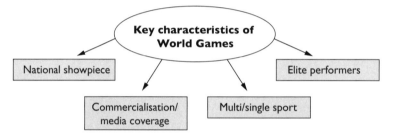

Organising your time

It is a good idea to make a revision timetable to ensure you use your time effectively. This should allow enough time to cover *all* the relevant material. However, it must also be realistic. For many students, revising for longer than an hour at a time becomes counter-productive, so allow for short relaxation breaks to refresh the body and mind.

Revision strategies

To revise a topic well, you should work carefully through your notes, using a copy of the specification to make sure you cover everything. Summarise your notes on the key points in each topic area. Topic cue cards with a summary of key facts and visual representations of the material (e.g. tables, spider diagrams, bubble diagrams) can be useful. These are easy to carry around for quick revision. Finally, use the Content Guidance and the Questions and Answers sections in this book. Discuss any problems or difficulties you have with your teachers or other students.

In many ways you should prepare for a unit test like an athlete prepares for a major event, such as the Olympic Games. An athlete trains every day for weeks or months before the big event, practising the required skills in order to achieve the best result on the day. So it is with exam preparation: everything you do should contribute to your chances of success in the unit test.

The following points summarise some of the strategies that you may wish to use to make sure your revision is as effective as possible:
- Use a revision timetable.
- Ideally, spend time revising in a quiet room, sitting upright at a desk or table, with no distractions.
- Test yourself regularly to assess the effectiveness of your revision. Ask yourself: 'Which techniques work best?' 'What are the gaps in my knowledge?' Remember to revise what you *don't* know.
- Practise past-paper questions to highlight gaps in your knowledge and understanding, and to improve your exam technique. You will also become familiar with the terminology used in exam questions.
- Spend some time doing 'active revision', such as:
  - discussing topics with fellow students and teachers
  - summarising your notes
  - compiling your own cue cards
  - answering previous test questions and self-checking against mark schemes
  - reading the sports pages, and watching the news and sports programmes

Revision progress

You may find it useful to keep track of your revision by drawing up a table for each topic. An example is shown below.

Complete column 2 to show how you have progressed with your revision:
- N = not yet revised
- P = partly revised
- F = fully revised

Complete column 3 to show how confident you are with the topic:
- 5 = high degree of confidence
- 1 = minimal confidence — practice questions were poorly answered

Topic: specialised training	Revised (N/P/F)	Self-evaluation (1–5)
Plyometrics		
PNF stretching		
Altitude training		
Glycogen loading		
Periodisation		
Lactate sampling/RER		

It is important to revise every topic, because any area of the specification could appear in the unit test.

The Unit 3 exam

The Unit 3 exam is divided into three sections matching the specification. In the exam, each section begins with a compulsory 14-mark question, which is marked according to 'banded statements'. The criteria in the bands link to the quality of written communication as well as to the number of relevant points you make. In addition to the compulsory question, in each section you are required to answer two from three questions, each worth 7 marks. You will have 2 hours to try to earn the 84 marks available. Unit 3 counts for 30% of your A-level (50% is awarded at AS and 20% is allocated to A2 coursework).

In the exam, it is important to write clearly in the spaces provided in the answer booklet. Avoid writing anything you want to be marked in the margins — the margins may be lost if papers are scanned for online marking.

There are a number of command words and terms commonly used in unit tests. It is important that you understand the meaning of each of these terms and that you answer the question appropriately

- **Analyse/critically evaluate/discuss** — put both sides of an argument or debate, stating your opinions as appropriate.
- **Apply/demonstrate knowledge** — use practical sporting examples to illustrate clearly your understanding of theoretical content.
- **Benefits** — positive outcomes.
- **Characteristics** — features or key distinguishing qualities.
- **Define** — give a clear, concise statement outlining what is meant by a particular term.
- **Describe** — give an accurate account of the main points in relation to the task set.
- **Explain** — give reasons to justify statements and opinions given in your answer.
- **State/give/list/identify** — show clear understanding of key characteristics.

Whatever the question style, you must read the wording carefully, underline or highlight key terms or phrases, think about your response and allocate time according to the number of marks available. Further advice and guidance on answering Unit 3 questions is provided in the Questions and Answers section of this guide.

Content
Guidance

Unit 3 is divided into three main topic areas:
- applied physiology to optimise performance
- psychological aspects that optimise performance
- evaluating contemporary issues and their influence on the performer

In the examination, each topic area has four questions: one compulsory extended-answer question and three further questions from which you must answer two.

This Content Guidance section summarises the key information that you need to understand and apply in the Unit 3 exam. It also includes useful examiner's tips and hints on 'What the examiner will expect you to be able to do'.

Remember that this Content Guidance is designed to support your revision and should be used in conjunction with your textbook, your own revision notes and other resources.

Applied physiology to optimise performance

Energy sources and systems

What the examiner will expect you to be able to do
- Identify where energy sources are located in the body and which energy source is used according to the intensity and duration of exercise.
- Explain how ATP is re-synthesised.
- Describe the ATP/PC system and the lactic acid system and their use in sporting situations.
- Describe the stages of the aerobic system, including Krebs cycle, the electron transport chain and the role of the mitochondria.
- Explain the lactate threshold through the energy continuum.

Adenosine triphosphate

Adenosine triphosphate (ATP) is the only usable form of energy in the body. The energy we derive from the foods that we eat, such as carbohydrates, has to be converted into ATP before the potential energy in them can be used. ATP consists of one molecule of adenosine and three phosphate groups:

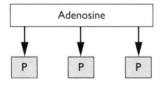

Energy is released by breaking down the bonds that hold ATP together. ATPase is the enzyme that breaks down ATP into ADP + P.

Sources of energy to replenish ATP
Phosphocreatine is used to re-synthesise ATP in the first 10 seconds of intense exercise. It is easy to break down and is stored in the muscle cells but stores of it are limited.

Food is also used for ATP re-synthesis. The main energy foods are:
- **Carbohydrates** — stored as **glycogen** in the muscles and the liver and converted into glucose during exercise. During high-intensity anaerobic exercise, glycogen can be broken down in the absence of oxygen, but it is broken down much more effectively during aerobic work when oxygen is present.

- **Fats** — stored as **triglycerides** and converted to free fatty acids when required. At rest, two-thirds of our energy requirements are met through the breakdown of fatty acids. This is because fat can produce more energy per gram than glycogen.
- **Protein** — approximately 5–10% of energy used during exercise comes from proteins in the form of amino acids. It tends to be used when stores of glycogen are low.

Carbohydrates and fats are the main energy providers and the intensity and duration of exercise play a major role in determining which of these are used. The breakdown of fats to free fatty acids requires more oxygen than the breakdown of glycogen, so during high-intensity exercise, when oxygen is in limited supply, glycogen will be the preferred source of energy. Fats, therefore, are the favoured fuel at rest and during long endurance-based activities.

Stores of glycogen are much smaller than stores of fat and it is important during prolonged periods of exercise not to deplete glycogen stores. Some glycogen needs to be conserved for later when the intensity could increase — for example, during the last kilometre of a marathon.

Energy systems

There are three energy systems that re-synthesise/replenish ATP:
- the **ATP-PC system**
- the **lactic acid system**
- the **aerobic system**

When deciding which is the predominant energy system in use, the two key words to consider are **intensity** and **duration**.

ATP-PC system

High-intensity activities lasting less than 10 seconds use predominantly the ATP-PC system. This system is anaerobic (no oxygen). Phosphocreatine is stored in the muscles and broken down to creatine and phosphate. Then energy is released for ATP re-synthesis. Aerobic energy is needed for this system to recover.

Advantages
- ATP can be re-synthesised rapidly using the ATP-PC system.
- Phosphocreatine stores can be re-synthesised quickly — (30 s = 50% replenishment and 3 min = 100%).
- There are no fatiguing by-products.
- It is possible to extend the time for the ATP-PC system through use of the creatine supplementation.

Disadvantages
- There is a limited supply of phosphocreatine in the muscle cell — it lasts for only 10 s.
- Only one mole of ATP can be re-synthesised through one mole of PC.

- PC re-synthesis can take place only in the presence of oxygen (i.e. the intensity of the exercise is reduced).

Lactic acid system

High-intensity activities with a duration of approximately 1 minute use mainly the lactic acid system. This system is anaerobic (no oxygen). In a process called **glycolysis**, glycogen is broken down into glucose, which is then broken down to pyruvic acid. In the absence of oxygen the pyruvic acid is converted to lactic acid and two molecules of ATP are produced.

Advantages
- ATP can be re-synthesised quite quickly because there are few chemical reactions.
- In the presence of oxygen, lactic acid can be converted back into liver glycogen or used as a fuel through oxidation into carbon dioxide and water.
- Can be used for a sprint finish (i.e. to produce an extra burst of energy).

Disadvantages
- Lactic acid is the by-product. The accumulation of acid in the body denatures enzymes and prevents them increasing the rate at which chemical reactions take place.

Aerobic system

Low-intensity activities with a duration of longer than 1–2 minutes use the aerobic system predominantly. This system uses oxygen. ATP is regenerated from glucose and fats in three stages:
- **Glycolysis** — glycogen is broken down into glucose, which is then broken down into pyruvic acid.
- **Krebs cycle** — the pyruvic acid diffuses into the matrix of the mitochondria and a complex cycle of reactions occurs. The reactions result in the production of two molecules of ATP plus carbon dioxide and hydrogen. The carbon dioxide is breathed out and the hydrogen is taken to the electron transport chain.
- **Electron transport chain** — the hydrogen given off in Krebs cycle is carried to the electron transport chain by hydrogen carriers. This occurs in the cristae of the mitochondria and the hydrogen splits into hydrogen ions and electrons. They are charged with potential energy. The hydrogen ions are oxidised to form water while the hydrogen electrons provide the energy to re-synthesise ATP. Throughout this process 34 molecules of ATP are formed.

Beta oxidation

Fats can also be used as an energy source in the aerobic system. They are broken down first into glycerol and then free fatty acids. These fatty acids undergo a process called beta oxidation whereby they are broken down in the mitochondria to generate acetyl-CoA, which is the entry molecule for the Krebs cycle. From this point on, fat metabolism follows the same path as carbohydrate (glycogen) metabolism. More ATP can be made from one mole of fatty acids than one mole of glycogen, which is why in long-duration exercise fatty acids will be the predominant energy source.

Advantages
- More ATP can be produced — 36 ATP molecules.
- There are no fatiguing by-products (only carbon dioxide and water).
- There are large stores of glycogen and triglyceride, so exercise can last a long time.

Disadvantages
- This is a complicated system. It takes a while for enough oxygen to become available to meet the demands of the activity and to ensure glycogen and fatty acids are completely broken down.
- Fatty acid transportation to muscles is low and requires 15% more oxygen to be broken down than glycogen.

The energy continuum

This refers to the continual movement from one energy system to another depending on the intensity and duration of the exercise. The ATP-PC/lactic acid threshold is the point at which the ATP-PC energy system is exhausted and the lactic acid system takes over. The lactic acid/aerobic threshold is the point at which the lactic acid system is exhausted and the aerobic system takes over. These thresholds can be highlighted in a graph.

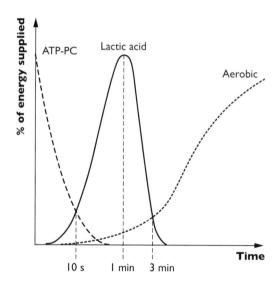

Maximising energy for ATP re-synthesis
By following an appropriate diet and training programme it is possible to enhance the production of energy from each of the energy systems.

Glycogen loading
This is a form of dietary manipulation involving maximising glycogen stores. Before an important competition, the performer eats a diet high in protein and fats for 3 days and exercises at relatively high intensity to burn off any existing carbohydrate stores.

This is followed by 3 days of a diet high in carbohydrates and some light training. This will greatly increase the stores of glycogen in the muscle.

The advantages are:
- increased glycogen synthesis
- increased glycogen stores in the muscle
- delayed onset of fatigue
- increase in endurance capacity

The disadvantages are:
- water retention, which results in bloating
- weight increase
- fatigue
- irritability during the depletion phase

Creatine monohydrate
This is a supplement used to increase the amount of phosphocreatine stored in the muscles. It allows the ATP-PC system to last longer and can help improve recovery times. Possible side-effects include dehydration and slight liver damage.

Soda loading
Drinking a solution of sodium bicarbonate increases the pH of the blood and makes it more alkaline. This increases the buffering capacity of the blood so it can neutralise the negative effects of lactic acid.

Training
This can improve the efficiency of each of the three energy systems, causing adaptations that will impact on ATP re-synthesis.

Causes of fatigue and the recovery process

What the examiner will expect you to be able to do
- Identify the causes of fatigue.
- Define 'oxygen deficit'.
- Define EPOC.
- Describe the fast and slow components of recovery.

Causes of fatigue

There are many causes of fatigue and these depend on the intensity and duration of the activity. For example, a marathon runner will fatigue through glycogen depletion whereas an 800 m runner will fatigue through lactic acid build-up.

Glycogen depletion

When glycogen stores are depleted athletes are said to 'hit the wall' as the body tries to metabolise fat but is unable to use this as a fuel on its own.

Lactic acid build-up

An accumulation of lactic acid releases hydrogen ions. These hydrogen ions cause an increase in the acidity of the blood plasma. This inhibits enzyme action and therefore the breakdown of glucose, and irritates nerve endings, causing pain.

Reduced rate of ATP synthesis

When stores of ATP and PC are depleted there is insufficient ATP to sustain muscular contractions.

Dehydration

Water is lost through sweating during exercise and if it is not replaced then dehydration occurs. Dehydration can have an effect on blood flow to the working muscles and results in a loss of electrolytes, such as calcium, which help with muscular contractions. Blood viscosity increases and blood pressure decreases. There is a reduction in sweating to prevent further water loss, which in turn increases core body temperature. This results in the performer being unable to meet the demands of the activity.

Reduced levels of calcium

For muscle contraction to occur there has to be a release of calcium. An increase in hydrogen ions (due to acid build-up) decreases the amount of calcium released.

Reduced levels of acetylcholine

This is a neurotransmitter that can help a nerve impulse to jump the synaptic cleft (the gap that separates the nerve ending from the muscle fibre) and initiate muscular contraction. When levels of acetylcholine are low the muscles become fatigued.

Thermoregulation

During exercise heat is generated in the body as a result of all the chemical reactions (metabolic processes) that take place to produce energy. Long-distance runners sometimes experience difficulty with temperature regulation. The heat produced through muscle contraction raises the core body temperature, which causes the blood viscosity to increase and metabolic processes to slow down. This means the performer is unable to sweat efficiently and dehydration occurs.

The thermoregulatory centre in the medulla oblongata controls temperature. Heat is transported to the surface of the skin by the blood and the vessels vasodilate, enabling heat to be lost through radiation, convection or the evaporation of sweat.

When the body is dehydrated, total blood volume decreases. More blood is redirected to the skin (to aid cooling), so the amount of blood and therefore oxygen available to the working muscles is reduced and this affects performance. In hot conditions this situation is exacerbated so it is important to acclimatise, enabling the body to modify the control systems that regulate blood flow to the skin and sweating.

The recovery process: EPOC

During recovery the body takes in increased amounts of oxygen. The oxygen is transported to the working muscles to maintain elevated rates of aerobic respiration. This surplus energy is used to help return the body to its pre-exercise state. This is known as excess post-exercise oxygen consumption (EPOC).

The oxygen debt

When we start to exercise insufficient oxygen is distributed to the tissues for all the energy production to be met aerobically, so the two anaerobic systems have to be used. The amount of oxygen that the subject was short of during the exercise is known as the **oxygen deficit**. This is compensated for by the surplus amount of oxygen — or oxygen debt — that results from EPOC.

The fast replenishment stage (alactacid component)

This involves the restoration of ATP and phosphocreatine stores and the re-saturation of myoglobin with oxygen. Elevated rates of respiration continue to supply oxygen to provide the energy for ATP production and phosphocreatine replenishment. Complete restoration of phosphocreatine takes up to 3 minutes but 50% of stores can be replenished after only 30 seconds, during which time approximately 2–3 litres of oxygen are consumed.

Myoglobin and replenishment of oxygen stores

Myoglobin has a high affinity for oxygen. It stores oxygen in the muscle and transports it from the capillaries to the mitochondria for energy provision. After exercise oxygen stores in the mitochondria are limited. The surplus of oxygen supplied through EPOC helps replenish these stores, taking up to 2 minutes and using approximately 0.5 litres of oxygen.

The slow replenishment stage (lactacid component)

This is concerned with the removal of lactic acid. It is the slower of the two processes and full recovery may take up to an hour, depending on the intensity and duration of the exercise. Lactic acid can be removed in four ways:

Destination	Approximate % lactic acid involved
Oxidation into carbon dioxide and water in the inactive muscles and organs	65
Conversion into glycogen — then stored in muscles/liver	20
Conversion into protein	10
Conversion into glucose	5

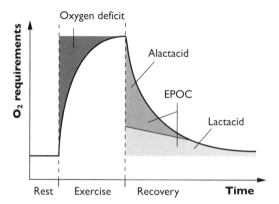

Glycogen replenishment

The replacement of glycogen stores depends on the type of exercise undertaken and when and how much carbohydrate is consumed following exercise. It may take several days to complete the restoration of glycogen after a marathon, but a significant amount of glycogen can be restored in less than an hour after long-duration, low-intensity exercise. Eating a high-carbohydrate meal will accelerate glycogen restoration, as will eating within an hour following exercise.

Increase in breathing and heart rates

This is important to assist in recovery where extra oxygen is required to return the body to its pre-exercise state. However, the increase in breathing and heart rates requires additional extra oxygen to provide energy for the muscles of the heart and respiratory system.

Increased activity of hormones

The continuation of sub-maximal exercise (such as a cool down) will keep hormone levels elevated and this will keep respiratory and metabolic levels high so that extra oxygen can be taken in.

Increase in body temperature

When temperature remains high, respiratory rate will also remain high and this will help the performer take in more oxygen during recovery. However, extra oxygen is needed to fuel this increase in temperature until the body returns to normal.

What makes a successful endurance performance?

What the examiner will expect you to be able to do

- Define VO_2 max and explain the factors that can affect it.
- Define OBLA and describe its effects.
- Understand the relationship between OBLA and VO_2 max.

VO$_2$ max and sporting performance

VO$_2$ max is the maximum volume of oxygen that can be taken in and used by the muscles per minute. A person's VO$_2$ max will determine endurance performance in sport.

Average VO$_2$ max values		
Female A-level PE student	Male A-level PE student	Paula Radcliffe
35–44 ml kg^{-1} min^{-1}	45–55 ml kg^{-1} min^{-1}	80 ml kg^{-1} min^{-1}

Evaluation of VO$_2$ max

There are various methods of evaluating VO$_2$ max:
- Douglas bag
- multi-stage fitness test
- Harvard step test
- PWC170 cycle ergometer test
- Cooper's 12-minute run

Factors affecting VO$_2$ max

Gender

A male endurance athlete will have a bigger VO$_2$ max (70 ml kg^{-1} min^{-1}) than a female endurance athlete (60 ml kg^{-1} min^{-1}). This is because the average female is smaller than the average male and females have:
- a smaller left ventricle and therefore a lower stroke volume
- a lower maximum cardiac output
- a lower blood volume resulting in lower haemoglobin levels
- lower tidal and ventilatory volumes

Age

As we get older our VO$_2$ max declines as our body systems become less efficient:
- maximum heart rate drops by around 5–7 beats per minute per decade
- an increase in peripheral resistance results in a decrease in maximal stroke volume
- blood pressure increases both at rest and during exercise
- less air is exchanged in the lungs due to a decline in vital capacity and an increase in residual air

Lifestyle

Smoking, sedentary lifestyle and poor diet can all reduce VO$_2$ max values.

Training

VO$_2$ max can be improved by up to 10–20% following a period of aerobic training (continuous, fartlek and aerobic interval) due to the following physiological adaptations:
- increased maximum cardiac output
- increased stroke volume/ejection fraction/cardiac hypertrophy
- greater heart rate range
- less oxygen being used for heart muscles, so more is available to other muscles
- increased A-VO$_2$ diff

- increased blood volume and haemoglobin/red blood cell/blood count
- increased stores of glycogen and triglycerides
- increased myoglobin (content of muscle)
- increased capillarisation (of muscle)
- increased number and size of mitochondria
- increased concentrations of oxidative enzymes
- increased lactate tolerance
- reduced body fat
- slow twitch hypertrophy

Body composition
Research has shown that VO_2 max decreases as percentage body fat increases.

Onset of blood lactate accumulation (OBLA)

Lactate is produced when hydrogen is removed from the lactic acid molecule. OBLA is the point at which lactate starts to rapidly accumulate in the blood. At rest, around 1–2 mmol l^{-1} lactic acid can be found in the blood. However, during intense exercise levels of lactic acid rise dramatically. OBLA occurs when the concentration of lactic acid is around 4 mmol l^{-1}.

OBLA gives an indication of endurance capacity. Some performers can work at higher levels of intensity than others before OBLA and can delay when the threshold occurs. OBLA is expressed as a percentage of VO_2 max. An average untrained person will work at about 50–60% of VO_2 max whereas a trained endurance performer can work at around 85–90% of VO_2 max before OBLA occurs.

Factors affecting the rate of lactate accumulation
Exercise intensity
High-intensity exercise increases the demand for energy (ATP). The fast twitch fibres used for high-intensity exercise can only maintain their workload with glycogen as the fuel. When glycogen is broken down in the absence of oxygen into pyruvic acid, lactic acid is formed.

Muscle fibre type
Slow twitch fibres produce less lactate than fast twitch fibres. When slow twitch fibres use glycogen as a fuel in the presence of oxygen, the glycogen can be broken down much more effectively and with little lactate production.

Rate of blood lactate removal
If the rate of lactate removal is equivalent to the rate of lactate production then the concentration of blood lactate remains constant. If lactate production increases then lactate will start to accumulate in the blood until OBLA is reached.

Training
Adaptations occur in trained muscles. Increased numbers of mitochondria and levels of myoglobin, together with an increase in capillary density, improve the capacity for aerobic respiration and therefore help to reduce the use of the lactic acid system.

Structure and function of muscles

What the examiner will expect you to be able to do
- Describe the structure and function of muscle.
- Identify the characteristics of the three fibre types: slow twitch (type 1), fast oxidative glycolytic (type IIa) and fast glycolytic (type IIb).
- Explain the sliding filament theory to include the structure of actin and myosin, the chemicals required to create movement and the process that occurs to create movement.
- Explain the terms 'motor units' and 'recruitment'.
- Explain muscle innervation.

Skeletal muscle is often referred to as voluntary, striped or striated muscle. Skeletal muscle is surrounded by a layer of connective tissue called the **epimysium**. This consists mainly of collagen fibres and its function is to provide a smooth surface for other muscles to glide against. Skeletal muscle is made up of bundles of muscle fibres, which are enclosed in a connective tissue sheath called the **perimysium**. Each of the individual muscle fibres is made up of many smaller fibres called myofibrils. Myofibrils are covered with a thin layer of connective tissue or **endomysium**.

The epimysium, perimysium and endomysium are all connected to one another so that when the muscle fibres contract, movement occurs through their links with the tendons and their attachment to bones at joints.

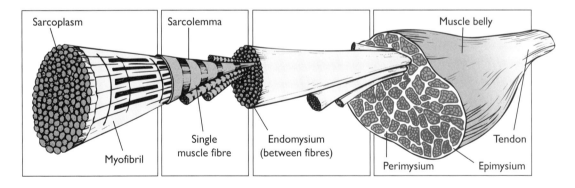

Control of muscular contraction

Muscle action has to be controlled in order for movement to be effective. There are several internal regulatory mechanisms that make this possible.
- **Proprioceptors** are sense organs in the muscles, tendons and joints that inform the body of the extent of movement that has taken place.
- **Muscle spindle apparatus** is made up of very sensitive proprioceptors that lie between skeletal muscle fibres. They provide information about the nature and

rate of change in muscle length. When the muscle stretches, the spindle also stretches and this sends an impulse to the spinal cord. If the muscle is stretched too far, the muscle spindle apparatus alters tension within the muscle, causing a stretch reflex which automatically shortens the muscle.

- **Golgi tendon organs** are thin pockets of connective tissue between the muscle fibre and tendon. They provide information to the central nervous system about the degree of tension or stretch in the muscle. When stretched, they trigger the reflex inhibition of the muscle that is contracting and stretching the tendon, and the reflex contraction of the antagonist muscle.

Types of muscle fibre

Three main types of muscle fibre can be identified:
- type I — slow oxidative
- type IIa — fast oxidative glycolytic
- type IIb — fast glycolytic

Our skeletal muscles contain all three types of fibre but not in equal proportions. The mix is mainly genetically determined. These fibres are grouped into motor units and only one type of fibre can be found in one particular unit.

The relative proportion of each fibre type varies in the same muscles of different people. For example, an elite endurance athlete will have a greater proportion of slow twitch fibres in the leg muscles than an elite sprinter who will have a greater proportion of fast twitch fibres. Postural muscles tend to have a greater proportion of slow twitch fibres as they are involved in maintaining body position for long periods of time.

All three fibre types have specific characteristics that allow them to perform their role successfully, as shown in the table below:

Characteristic	Type I	Type IIa	Type IIb
Contraction speed (ms^{-1})	slow (10)	fast (50)	fast (50)
Motor neurone size	small	large	large
Force produced	low	high	high
Fatiguability	low	medium	high
Mitochondrial density	high	medium	low
Myoglobin content	high	medium	low
Glycogen store	low	high	high
Triglyceride store	high	medium	low
Capillary density	high	medium	low
Aerobic capacity	high	medium	low
Anaerobic capacity	low	medium	high

The sliding filament theory

A myofibril is the contractile unit of the muscle. It runs the length of the fibre. Under a microscope it is possible to see cross-bands or striations across it.

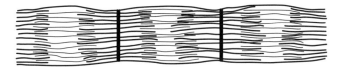

This pattern of cross-banding is repeated along the length of the myofibril. The repeated unit is called a **sarcomere**. Each sarcomere contains two types of protein filament: the thick myosin filaments and the thin actin filaments. During contraction, these slide across one another and connect or make **crossbridges**. This overlapping creates the striped appearance of the sarcomere.

A sarcomere is constructed as follows:

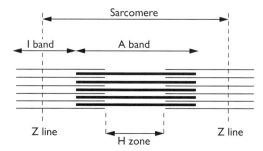

The A bands contain both actin and myosin filaments. The I bands contain only actin filaments and the H zones contain only myosin filaments. When the muscle contracts, the Z lines move closer together, the width of the I bands and H zones decreases while the A band stays the same.

The actin has binding sites and the myosin can attach to these through tiny protein projections that look similar to golf clubs. Each of these projections contains ATPase, the enzyme used to break down ATP, which provides the energy to bind the myosin crossbridge onto the actin filament and allow muscular contraction to take place.

The actin filament also contains two molecules called **troponin** and **tropomyosin**. These cover the binding sites of the actin and prevent crossbridges from forming. This can be overcome by the release of calcium from the sarcoplasmic reticulum, which attracts the troponin, neutralises the tropomyosin and releases the binding sites on the actin, allowing crossbridges to occur.

The sliding filaments are believed to work rather like a ratchet mechanism where the crossbridges constantly attach, detach then reattach with the net result of shortening the sarcomere.

The motor unit

Muscle innervation occurs when an impulse travels from the cerebrum or spinal cord. Impulses travel along nerves to the muscle. A motor unit comprises one motor neurone and its corresponding muscle fibres.

One motor neurone cannot stimulate the whole muscle. Instead a motor neurone will stimulate a number of fibres (between 15 and 2000) within that muscle. Each motor unit contains only one kind of muscle fibre, for example only slow oxidative fibres.

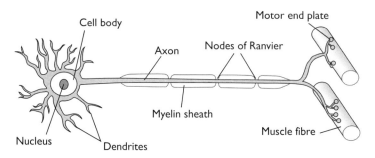

The all-or-none law

A minimum amount of stimulation — the **threshold** — is required to start a contraction. If an impulse is equal to or more than the threshold then all the muscle fibres in a motor unit will contract. If the impulse is less than the threshold then no muscle action will occur. As such, the motor unit exhibits an all-or-none response.

Gradation of contraction

This refers to the strength or force exerted by a muscle. It depends on the following factors.

Recruitment

If more motor units are recruited, more muscle fibres contract, increasing the force that can be produced. This is also referred to as **multiple unit summation**.

Frequency

The greater the frequency of stimuli, the greater the tension developed by the muscle. If the stimuli occur infrequently, the calcium concentration in the sarcomere returns to resting levels before the arrival of the next stimulus (S). When the stimuli occur frequently, not all the calcium released in response to the first stimulus is taken back into the sarcoplasmic reticulum. As a result summation occurs. This is also called **wave summation**, where repeated activation of a motor neurone stimulating a given muscle fibre results in summation.

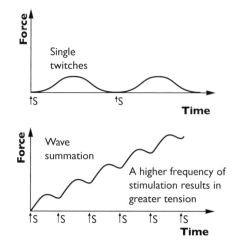

Timing
If all the motor units are stimulated at exactly the same time, maximum force can be applied. This is referred to as **spatial summation** or **synchronisation**.

Sports supplements and ergogenic aids

What the examiner will expect you to be able to do
- For each supplement and ergogenic aid, explain what it is, discuss the advantages and disadvantages of its use, and identify which athletes use it.
- Explain how to prepare the body for training and performance through water and electrolyte balance, diet and achieving optimal weight.
- Explain how this is achieved for different performers, such as endurance and power athletes.

Types of supplement

Sports supplements are used to increase energy stores, which in turn enhance athletic performance.

Creatine monohydrate
This increases the amount of phosphocreatine stored in the muscles, which allows the ATP-PC system to last longer and can help improve recovery times. Athletes in explosive events, such as sprinting, are likely to experience most benefit. Possible side-effects include dehydration, bloating, muscle cramps and slight liver damage.

Herbal remedies
These are often advertised as 'natural' products that have effects ranging from decreasing body fat to elevating blood testosterone levels, increasing muscle mass, enhancing energy, improving strength and stamina, and generally improving health and athletic performance. Many of these claims are unfounded and care should be taken by athletes who use them. Common remedies include electrolyte stamina tablets for athletes who experience a lot of fluid loss, whey protein powder to increase muscle metabolism, gotu kola powder to enhance mental alertness and ginseng to increase endurance and enhance muscle recovery.

Protein supplements
These are used to enhance muscle repair and growth. This can increase endurance and increase or maintain muscle mass. Protein supplements are often taken by strength athletes, who believe that protein is important to build muscle and to repair muscle that is broken down during strenuous exercise. However, a diet high in protein can put a strain on the liver and kidneys and may cause a negative nitrogen balance, which slows down muscle growth and can cause fatigue.

Sodium bicarbonate
Drinking a solution of sodium bicarbonate reduces the acidity in the muscle cells. This delays fatigue and allows the performer to continue exercising at high intensity for

longer. Sodium bicarbonate increases the buffering capacity of the blood, so neutralising the negative effects of lactic acid. However, it can also result in vomiting, pain, cramping, diarrhoea or a feeling of being bloated. Athletes who use the lactic acid system, such as 400 m runners, produce a lot of acidity so will benefit from 'soda loading'.

Caffeine

Caffeine is a stimulant so it can increase mental alertness and reduce fatigue. It is also thought to improve the mobilisation of fatty acids in the body, thereby sparing muscle glycogen stores. It is used by endurance performers, who predominantly use the aerobic system, because fats are the preferred fuel for low-intensity, long-duration exercise. The drawbacks of caffeine are the increased risk of dehydration (it is a diuretic), irritability, insomnia and anxiety.

Glycogen loading

This is a form of dietary manipulation designed to maximise muscle glycogen stores. It is often used by long-distance runners to prevent them 'hitting the wall'. It increases glycogen synthesis, increases glycogen stores in the muscle, delays fatigue and increases endurance capacity. The disadvantages can be water retention, heavy legs, weight increase and, during the depletion phase, irritability.

Ergogenic aids

All athletes want to improve their performance. Substances that improve performance are called **ergogenic aids**. The following are illegal ergogenic aids.

- **Anabolic steroids** (artificially produced hormones) promote muscle growth, strength and lean body weight. Power athletes such as sprinters might want to use them. Side-effects include liver damage, heart and immune system problems, acne and behavioural changes such as aggression, paranoia and mood swings.
- **Human growth hormone (HGH)** is an artificially produced hormone that can increase muscle mass and decrease fat. It is used by a range of athletes such as sprinters, rugby players and even endurance performers. The full extent of its use is unknown because it is hard to detect in the blood. HGH use can lead to diseases of the heart and nerves, glucose intolerance, and high levels of blood fats.
- **Beta blockers** are used to decrease anxiety. They can improve accuracy in precision sports by steadying the nerves. Snooker players and golfers might want to use them. The Professional Golfers' Association announced in 2007 that members would be tested for use of beta blockers, but this decision was controversially withdrawn at the 2008 British Open. Side-effects include tiredness due to low blood pressure and slower heart rate, which affects aerobic capacity.
- **Erythropoietin (EPO)** is a natural hormone produced by the kidneys. It can be manufactured artificially. It increases haemoglobin levels, which improves the oxygen-carrying capacity of the blood and this can increase the amount of work performed. EPO tends to be used by endurance performers who need effective oxygen transport. Use of EPO can result in blood clotting, stroke and, in a few cases, death.

Preparing the body for training and performance

Water and electrolyte balance

When you undertake exercise, energy is required and some of that energy is released as heat. Sweating prevents you from overheating but water is lost from the body during this cooling process. Once the body starts to lose water during exercise, a drop in blood volume can result. When this occurs, the heart has to work harder to move blood around the body and less oxygen is available to the working muscles. This will affect performance. It is therefore important to drink early and often when exercising.

Electrolytes dissolve in water and any water loss through sweating can change the electrolyte balance. The balance of the electrolytes in our bodies is important for the normal functioning of cells and organs. Common electrolytes include sodium, potassium and chloride ions. These are essential for the electrical transmission of nerve impulses that control muscle contraction.

Achieving optimal weight

The most accurate weight assessments look at body composition. This means calculating the percentage of body fat and lean body mass. Women should have no more than 30% body fat, men no more than 20% body fat.

Optimal weight in sport varies according to activity. Training and dietary choice affect the amount of muscle mass and body fat. A prop in rugby league will be heavier than a winger because the requirements of these positions are different — props need a large muscle mass to support the scrum whereas wingers need to be leaner since they need speed to evade the opposition. In boxing, optimal weight is crucial to keep in a certain weight category, while a jockey needs to be light, as excess weight is seen as a handicap.

Athletes' diets

Nutrition and diet can contribute to a successful performance. A balanced diet is essential for optimum performance in all sporting activities and should contain 10–15% protein, 20–25% fats and 60–75% carbohydrates.

Diet composition of endurance versus power athletes

The body's preferred fuel for any endurance sport is muscle glycogen. If muscle glycogen breakdown exceeds its replacement, then glycogen stores become depleted. This results in fatigue and the inability to maintain the duration and intensity of training. In order to replenish and maintain glycogen stores, endurance athletes need a diet rich in carbohydrates. Research suggests that endurance athletes need to consume at least 6–10g carbohydrate per kilogram of body weight per day. Some endurance athletes manipulate their diet to maximise aerobic energy production. One method is glycogen loading (see page 15).

Water is another key nutrient for endurance athletes (see above).

Proteins are very important for power athletes. Insufficient protein will lead to muscle breakdown as proteins are important for tissue growth and repair.

Specialised training

What the examiner will expect you to be able to do
- Explain what each type of training discussed below involves, the physiological reasons for its use, which athletes find it useful and whether it is effective.

Altitude training

Altitude training is used to improve endurance performance. The percentage of oxygen in the air is the same at sea level and at altitude. However, the **partial pressure** of oxygen decreases as altitude increases, causing a reduction in the diffusion gradient between the air and the lungs and between the alveoli and the blood. As a result, haemoglobin is not fully saturated at altitude, which results in a lower oxygen-carrying capacity of the blood. As less oxygen is delivered to working muscles, fatigue sets in earlier. This leads to a decrease in performance (of aerobic activities).

Altitude training enhances oxygen transport due to an increase in the number of red blood cells and haemoglobin levels resulting from an increase in the hormone erythropoietin. Altitude training also has some disadvantages:
- expense
- altitude sickness
- difficulties of training due to the lack of oxygen
- detraining — training intensity has to reduce when the performer first trains at altitude because less oxygen is available
- benefits are quickly lost on return to sea level

Plyometrics

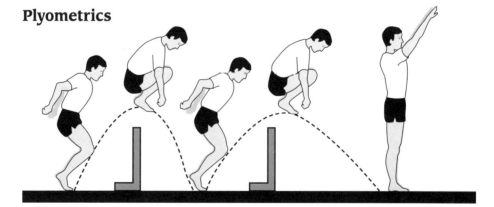

If leg power is crucial to successful performance, for example in long jump, 100 m sprint or rebounding in basketball, this method of strength training improves power or elastic strength. It is based on the concept that muscles generate more force if they have previously been stretched. This occurs in plyometrics when, on landing, the muscle performs an eccentric contraction (lengthens under tension). This stimulates the muscle spindle apparatus as it detects the rapid lengthening of the muscle and then sends nerve impulses to the central nervous system (CNS). If the CNS perceives that the muscle is lengthening too quickly, it will initiate a stretch reflex, causing a powerful concentric contraction as the performer jumps up.

To develop arm strength, performers could do press-ups with mid-air claps or practise throwing and catching a medicine ball.

PNF stretching

Proprioceptive neuromuscular facilitation (PNF) is an advanced stretching technique. It is considered to be one of the most effective forms of flexibility training for increasing range of motion since it facilitates muscular inhibition. First, the muscle should be passively stretched, then contracted isometrically against a resistance while in a stretched position for a period of at least 10 seconds. When it is passively stretched again there is an increase in the range of motion. PNF stretching tends to be more effective with the help of a partner.

(a)

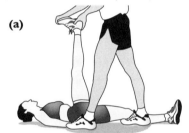

The individual performs a passive stretch with the help of a partner and extends the leg until tension is felt. The stretch is detected by the muscle spindles. If the muscle is being stretched too far then a stretch reflex should occur.

(b)

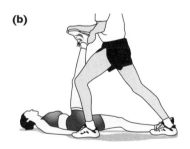

The individual then isometrically contracts the muscle for at least 10 seconds by pushing his/ her leg against the partner who supplies just enough resistance to hold the leg in a stationary position. Golgi tendon organs are sensitive to tension developed in a muscle. During an isometric contraction they send an inhibitory signal, which overrides the excitatory signal from the muscle spindle and delays the stretch reflex.

(c)

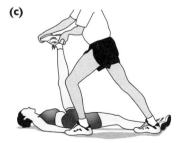

There is further relaxation of the target muscle and it can be stretched further during the next passive stretch

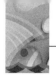

Periodisation

Periodisation involves dividing the year into periods when specific training occurs.

The **macrocycle** involves a long-term performance goal. For a footballer it may be the length of the season; for an athlete it could be 4 years building up to the Olympic Games. The macrocycle is made up of three distinct periods:
• preparation period/pre-season training
• competition period
• transition or recovery period

The **mesocycle** describes a short-term goal (2–8 weeks) within the macrocycle. The focus may be a component of fitness — for example, power, reaction time or speed for a sprinter, strength endurance or cardio-respiratory endurance for an endurance performer.

The **microcycle** normally represents 1 week of training repeated throughout the mesocycle (what the performer does from Monday to Sunday, including rest days, usually in a 3:1 ratio).

The **training unit** is a description of one training session, which will follow a key training objective.

Tapering and peaking

Many elite performers maintain a high level of fitness throughout the season but a few days before a big competition they reduce their daily training loads. This is called **tapering**. Timing a season so that full mental and physical preparation occurs just before a major event is called **peaking**.

Double periodisation

Some sports require an athlete to peak more than once in a season. A long-distance athlete, for example, may want to peak in winter during the cross-country season and again in the summer on the track. An international footballer may want to peak for an important cup final for his club and for a cup competition later in the year for his country. These performers have to follow a **double-periodised** year.

Lactate sampling

Elite performers in sports such as running, swimming and rowing use blood lactate measurements to monitor training and predict performance. The measurements are used to rate training intensity — the higher the pace at which the lactate threshold occurs, the fitter the athlete is considered to be. Lactate sampling allows the performer to select relevant training zones — expressed in terms of heart rate (beats per minute) or power (watts) — in order to get the desired training effect. Regular lactate testing provides a comparison from which the coach and performer can see whether improvement has occurred. If test results show a lactate increase, this indicates that the performer has increased peak speed or power, lengthened time to exhaustion, improved recovery heart rate and achieved a higher lactate threshold.

Respiratory exchange ratio (RER)

Energy sources such as carbohydrates, fat and protein can all be oxidised to produce energy. For a certain volume of oxygen, the energy released will depend on the energy source. Calculating the RER will determine which energy source is being oxidised. RER is the ratio of carbon dioxide produced to oxygen consumed and is also referred to as the **respiratory quotient** (RQ).

- an RER of 0.7 indicates that the predominant energy source is fats
- an RER between 0.7 and 1.0 indicates a mix of carbohydrate and fats as the main energy source
- an RER greater than 1.0 indicates anaerobic respiration since more carbon dioxide is being produced than oxygen consumed

Sports injuries

What the examiner will expect you to be able to do
- Explain how injuries can be prevented and discuss rehabilitation.
- Explain what hyperbaric chambers, oxygen tents and ice baths are.
- Identify the physiological reasons for their use.
- Discuss which athletes find them useful.
- Decide whether they are effective measures.
- Define delayed onset of muscle soreness (DOMS) and explain why it occurs.

Prevention of injuries

Proper preparation before exercise can reduce injuries by up to 25%. Injuries can be prevented by:
- using the correct equipment, for example mouth guards or pads if required
- wearing correct clothing, for example trainers with good friction and support
- using training methods that allow for rest days
- including warm-ups and cool-downs in training sessions

Specialised rehabilitation techniques

Hyperbaric chambers

The aim of hyperbaric chambers is to reduce the recovery time for an injury. The chamber is pressurised and in some chambers a mask is worn. The pressure increases the amount of oxygen that can be breathed in, which means more oxygen can be diffused to the injured area. The dissolved oxygen reduces swelling and stimulates the body's cells to repair.

Oxygen tents

Oxygen tents are also known as **hypoxic tents**. Elite sportsmen and sportswomen may sleep in them overnight — the tents simulate the effects of high altitude by

content guidance

providing a low-oxygen environment. The oxygen depletion causes production of higher levels of haemoglobin, which means more oxygen can be extracted from the blood for extra energy. Oxygen tents do not make a difference to the speed of the healing process, but do mean that when the performer has recovered from injury, he or she will have retained a level of fitness that allows him or her to return to sport almost immediately. The tents are useful for endurance activities such as cycling, and sports that require a high level of stamina such as football.

Ice baths

After a hard training session or match, sports performers may get into an ice bath for 5–10 minutes. The cold water causes the blood vessels to tighten and drains the blood from the legs. The blood takes with it the lactic acid that has built up during the activity. On leaving the bath, the legs fill up with fresh blood, which invigorates the muscles with oxygen to help the cells function better.

Delayed onset of muscle soreness (DOMS)

One aim of training is to improve fitness levels. An individual who wants to improve strength may work at higher intensities to overload the muscle and stimulate muscle hypertrophy. When this occurs the individual may experience painful muscles some 24–48 hours after exercise. This is called **delayed onset of muscle soreness**.

The muscle soreness is a result of structural damage to muscle fibres and connective tissue surrounding the fibres. DOMS usually occurs following excessive eccentric contraction when muscle fibres are put under a lot of strain. This type of muscular contraction is performed mostly during weight training and plyometrics.

A thorough warm-up and cool-down can help to avoid the delayed soreness or at least keep it to a minimum. If eccentric muscle contractions are the major causal factors, training should minimise their use and increase intensity gradually.

Mechanics of movement

What the examiner will expect you to be able to do
- Use vectors and scalars in relation to acceleration, momentum and impulse in sprinting.
- Describe Newton's laws and apply them to movements.
- Explain the application of forces in sporting activities.
- Describe projectile motion, including the factors affecting distance and vector components of parabolic flight.
- Explain the concept of angular motion and how it is conserved during flight.
- Describe the moment of inertia and explain its relationship with angular velocity.

Newton's laws of motion

Newton's first law

A body will continue in its state of rest or motion in a straight line unless compelled to change that state by external forces exerted upon it.

For example, in a penalty, the ball (body) will remain on the spot (state of rest) until it is kicked by the player (an external force is exerted upon it).

Newton's second law

The rate of change of momentum of a body (or the acceleration for a body of constant mass) is proportional to the force causing it and the change that takes place in the direction in which the force acts.

For example, when a player kicks (force applied) the ball during a game, the acceleration of the ball (rate of change of momentum) is proportional to the size of the force. So, the harder the ball is kicked, the further and faster it will go.

Newton's third law

To every action there is an equal and opposite reaction.

For example, when a footballer jumps up (action) to win a header, a force is exerted on the ground in order to gain height. At the same time the ground exerts an upward force (equal and opposite reaction) upon the footballer.

Measurements used in linear motion

Linear motion is motion in a straight or curved line, with all body parts moving the same distance at the same speed in the same direction.

The measurements used in linear motion are:
- **mass**, a physical quantity expressing the amount of matter in a body — our mass is made up of bone, muscle, fat, tissue and fluid and is measured in kilograms
- **weight** — the force on a given mass due to gravity
- **inertia** — the resistance an object has to a change in its state of motion
- **distance** — the length of the path a body follows when moving from one position to another
- **displacement** — the length of a straight line joining the start and finish points
- **speed** — the rate of change of position, which can be calculated as follows:

$$\text{speed (m s}^{-1}) = \frac{\text{distance covered (m)}}{\text{time taken (s)}}$$

- **velocity** — the rate of change of displacement is a **vector quantity**. This is a more precise description of motion and can be calculated as follows:

$$\text{velocity (m s}^{-1}) = \frac{\text{distance covered (m)}}{\text{time taken (s)}}$$

- **acceleration** and **deceleration** — refer to the rate of change of velocity
- **momentum** — the product of the mass and velocity of an object

These measurements can be split into two groups:
- **Scalar quantities** are described in terms of size or magnitude — mass, inertia, distance and speed are scalar quantities.
- **Vector quantities** are described in terms of size and direction — weight, acceleration, deceleration, displacement, velocity and momentum are vector quantities.

Forces and vectors

Force is a vector quantity. Remember, a vector has size and direction. Both vertical and horizontal forces act upon sports performers.

Vertical forces
- **Weight** (W) is a gravitational force that the Earth exerts on a body, pulling it towards the centre of the Earth (or, effectively, downwards).
- **Reaction** (R) occurs whenever two bodies are in contact with one another.

Horizontal forces
- **Friction** (F) occurs when two bodies in contact with each other have a tendency to slip or slide over each other. Friction acts in opposition to motion.
- **Air resistance** (AR) opposes the motion of a body travelling through the air. Air resistance is often referred to as 'drag'. It depends on the velocity, cross-section, shape and surface characteristics of the moving body. The degree of drag depends on the factors listed above and on the type of fluid environment through which the body is travelling. Compare running in water with running on land: there is a much greater drag force in water due to its greater density.

Free-body diagrams
For your exam you need to know how forces are applied in sporting activities. You can show the forces acting on a body as arrows in free-body diagrams. The length of the arrow reflects the size of the force.

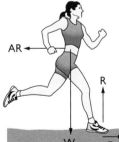

- The weight force (W) is always drawn down from the centre of mass.
- The reaction force (R) starts from where two bodies are in contact with one another. This contact can be between the foot and the ground or between sports equipment and a ball e.g. a tennis racket and a tennis ball.
- The friction force (F) starts from where two bodies are in contact and is opposite to the direction of any potential slipping. It is usually drawn in the same direction as motion.
- Air resistance (AR) is drawn from the centre of mass and opposes the direction of motion of the body.

Net force is the resultant force acting on a body when all other forces have been considered. Net force is often discussed in terms of balanced versus unbalanced forces.

A **balanced force** is when two or more forces acting on a body are equal in size but opposite in direction. If there is zero net force, there is no change in the state of motion.

An **unbalanced force** is when a force acting in one direction on a body is larger than the force acting in the opposite direction.

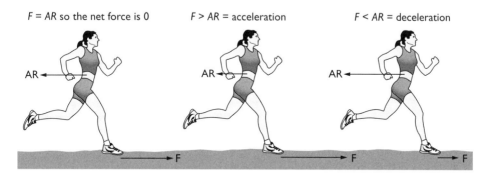

Impulse

Impulse is the product of the average size of the force acting on a body and the time for which that force is applied. It is equivalent to the change in momentum. In a sporting environment, impulse can be used to add speed to a body or object, or to slow it down on impact. It can be calculated as follows:

impulse (newton seconds/N s) = force × time

Impulse can be represented by a force–time graph. The graphs below show various stages of a 100 m sprint. It is important to note that in running or sprinting, positive impulse occurs for acceleration at take-off, whereas negative impulse occurs when the foot lands to provide a braking action.

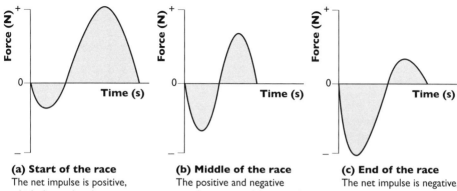

(a) Start of the race
The net impulse is positive, which shows that the sprinter is accelerating

(b) Middle of the race
The positive and negative impulses are equal (net impulse zero), which means that there is no acceleration or deceleration, so the sprinter is running at a constant velocity

(c) End of the race
The net impulse is negative, which shows that the sprinter is decelerating

Projectile motion

This refers to the motion of either an object or the human body being 'projected' into the air at an angle. Three factors determine the horizontal distance that a projectile can travel:

- angle of release
- height of release
- velocity of release

Forces affecting projectiles

Weight and air resistance are two forces that affect projectiles while they are in the air. Projectiles with a large weight have a small air resistance and follow a parabolic flight path.

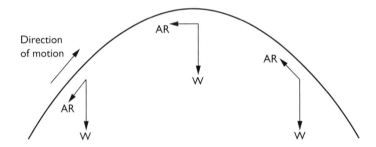

The forces acting on the flight path of a shot put. The shot has a large mass so the weight arrow is longer than the air resistance arrow.

Air resistance has a much greater effect on projectiles with a lighter mass, such as a shuttlecock, and this causes them to deviate from the parabolic pathway.

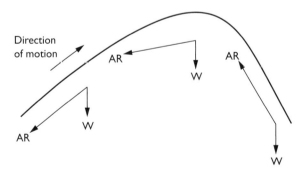

The forces acting on the flight path of a shuttlecock. Compared with the shot, the shuttlecock has a lighter mass and an unusual shape, which increases its air resistance. In a serve the shuttlecock starts off with a high velocity, provided by the force of the racket. As the shuttle continues its flight path, it slows down and the effect of air resistance decreases.

Angular momentum

Axes of rotation

There are three axes of rotation:

- the transverse axis runs from side to side across the body, as seen in a somersault
- the frontal axis runs from front to back, as seen in a cartwheel
- the longitudinal axis runs from top to bottom, as seen in a spinning ice skater

Angular momentum is rotation. It involves an object or body in motion around an axis. It depends on the **moment of inertia** and **angular velocity**. These two quantities are inversely proportional — if the moment of inertia increases, angular velocity decreases, and vice versa.

Moment of inertia is the resistance of a body to angular motion (rotation). This depends on the mass of the body and the distribution of mass around the axis. The closer the mass is to the axis of rotation, the easier it is to turn — so the moment of inertia is low. Increasing the distance of the distribution of mass from the axis of rotation will increase the moment of inertia.

Angular momentum is a conserved quantity — it remains constant unless an external torque (force) acts upon it (Newton's first law). For example, when a figure-skater performs a spin, turning on a longitudinal (vertical) axis, there is no change in his angular momentum until he uses his blades to slow the spin down.

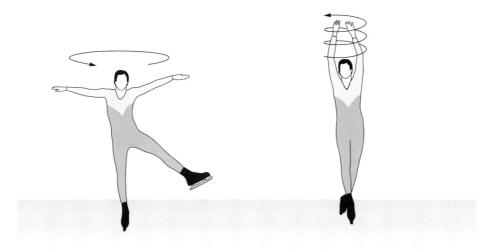

Ice is an almost friction-free surface so there is very little resistance to movement. The figure skater can manipulate his moment of inertia to increase or decrease the speed of the spin. At the start of the spin his arms and leg are outstretched. This increases their distance from the axis of rotation, resulting in a large moment of inertia and a large angular momentum in order to start the spin (rotation is therefore slow).

When the figure skater brings his arms and legs back in line with the rest of his body, the distance of these body parts to the axis of rotation decreases significantly. This reduces the moment of inertia, meaning that angular momentum has to increase. The result is a very fast spin (i.e. angular velocity increases).

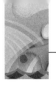

Psychological aspects that optimise performance

Personality

> **What the examiner will expect you to be able to do**
> - Give a clear definition of personality.
> - Describe the three approaches to personality.
> - Discuss profiles of mood states.
> - Evaluate personality testing using correct terminology and examples.
> - Describe characteristics of NACH and NAF performers.
> - Describe the personality and situational characteristics relating to them, with examples. Note the links with attribution theory and self-confidence.

Personality is defined as the unique, psychological and behavioural features of an individual.

Interactionist perspective

The interactionist approach suggests that personality is made up of traits and the influence of environmental experiences. It accepts that traits and social learning are relevant and combines them. The equation to describe this is:

$$B = f(P \times E)$$

This means that behaviour (B) is a function (f) of personality traits (P) and the environment (E). Performers adapt to the situation. For instance, a generally introverted rhythmic gymnast displays extroverted characteristics to appeal to the judges during a competition.

Trait perspective

Trait theory suggests that we are born with certain personality characteristics, which are determined genetically. These characteristics are likely to be shown in all situations, so behaviour can be predicted. Trait psychologists suggest that personality is stable and enduring. For instance, a netballer who is calm and controlled will remain so even when playing against an opponent who is continually making contact with her. The coach will be confident that this player will not lash out. The trait approach does not consider the effects that environmental learning may have on the performer, or that people may consciously decide to structure their own personalities. This illustrates the nature (trait) versus nurture (social learning) debate.

Eysenck's model

Eysenck suggested that an individual's personality lies on two continua: between extroversion and introversion, and between stability and neurosis.

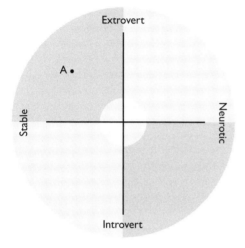

Extrovert	Introvert
• Likes social situations • Outgoing • Likes performing to an audience • Becomes bored easily as reticular activating system (RAS) is not easily stimulated	• Dislikes social situations • Reserved • Dislikes performing to an audience • Easily over-aroused as RAS is highly stimulated
Stable	**Neurotic**
• Reliable • Consistent • Calm	• Unpredictable • Restless • Volatile

The four quadrants in Eysenck's model are used to describe an individual's personality. For example, a stable extrovert (performer A in the diagram above) is even-tempered and outgoing, while a stable introvert is consistent and reserved. A neurotic extrovert is ill-tempered and lively, while a neurotic introvert is unpredictable and shy.

Narrow band theory

This theory also suggests that personality is innate. It groups personality into two types.

Type A	Type B
• High stress/arousal level • Competitive • Lacks tolerance • Needs to be in control of the task • Fast worker	• Low stress/arousal level • Not concerned with competition • Patient • Does not need to be in control of the task • Works slowly

Tip Candidates often omit narrow band theory from answers on the three approaches to personality — make sure you include it.

Social learning perspective

This approach suggests that personality is not innate but is learned from our experiences. It changes according to the situation, so behaviour cannot be predicted. We observe and copy the behaviour and personality of significant others, such as parents, peers, coaches and role models in the media. Socialisation also plays an important part. If behaviour is successful or is praised, it is likely that we will imitate it. For instance, if a tennis coach praises a player for showing determination and controlled emotions during matches, her team-mates will copy the behaviour to gain the same reinforcement. A performer is more likely to copy the behaviour and personality of people who share characteristics such as gender, age and ability level.

Personality testing

Methods used to measure personality and predict behaviour include observation, questionnaires such as profile of mood states (POMS), and biological testing, for instance heart-rate monitoring. However, testing has proved inconclusive and as yet there is no certain method of linking personality with sport or behaviour.

Observation is a real-life method whereby a performer's behaviour is analysed before, during and after play. Questionnaires are a cheap and quick method of gaining a vast amount of information. Biological tests generate factual data on physiological responses such as stress levels but necessitate the performer wearing a monitor, which may be restrictive.

Limitations of personality testing

Personality testing has been relatively unsuccessful because results are often vague. Performers may change their behaviour if they know they are being tested or observed — for instance, they may be inhibited if they have to play while wearing a heart-rate monitor. This immediately gives unreliable results. Performers may not give truthful answers on questionnaires, again lowering reliability. Interpreting the behaviour of a performer during observations is subjective — different testers may not see behaviour in the same light and results can lack objectivity. To be reliable, the results of a test should be the same when the test is repeated.

Tests can also lack external and ecological validity. This means they cannot be generalised to the wider population. How people act while playing sport may not be how they act on a day-to-day basis. There is little evidence to support the idea of a 'sporty' personality type or that certain personality types are suited to specific activities. For example, not all team-sport players are extroverts, neither are all long-distance runners introverts. All personality types should be encouraged to participate in a variety of sports, so increasing the number of people leading active lifestyles. No performer should be excluded from participation based on their personality.

Profile of mood states (POMS)

The POMS was designed to measure the moods of sports performers. Levels of tension, depression, anger, vigour, fatigue and confusion of both successful and unsuccessful performers have been profiled. Results show that successful performers generate an 'iceberg profile' (named after its shape). This is based on a high score for the positive mood (i.e. vigour) and a low score for negative mood states, as shown below.

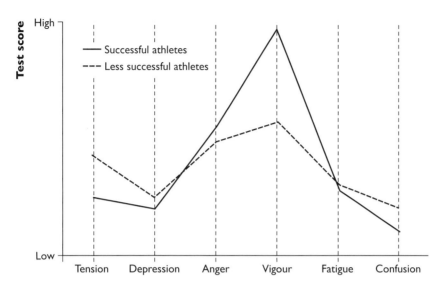

Research has shown that many, but not all, elite athletes exhibit such a profile. The question arises whether successful performers had the profile *before* they became elite, or was the profile a *result* of becoming elite?

> **Tip** When discussing POMS and evaluating personality testing, make sure that your examples relate specifically to personality — trait, social learning and interactionist perspectives are also seen in leadership and aggression.

Achievement motivation

Atkinson and McClelland suggested that, in demanding situations, performers exhibit either **need to achieve** (NACH) or **need to avoid failure** (NAF) characteristics. The characteristic displayed depends on the performer's personality and on the situation. It dictates the level of competitiveness shown by the individual.

NACH performer	NAF performer
Exhibits approach behaviour	Exhibits avoidance behaviour
Has high self-efficacy/confidence	Has low self-efficacy/confidence
Enjoys challenges	Dislikes challenges
Will take risks	Will take the easy option
Sticks with the task until it is complete	Gives in easily, especially if failing
Regards failure as a step to success	
Welcomes feedback and uses it to improve	Does not welcome feedback
Takes personal responsibility for the outcome	May experience learned helplessness
Attributes success internally	Attributes failure internally
Likes an audience when performing	Dislikes performing in front of an audience

NACH performer	NAF performer
Very competitive — likes tasks with • a low probability of success (i.e. a challenging task) • a high incentive (i.e. will be extremely proud to have achieved his/her goal)	Is not competitive — likes tasks with • a high probability of success (i.e. an easy task) • a low incentive (i.e. little satisfaction in achieving his/her goal)
An example of a NACH performer is a snowboarder who decides to take the risky black off-piste route rather than the easier run down the mountain, knowing she is likely to fall, but seeing it as a challenge	An example of a NAF performer is a mid-table squash player who prefers to play opponents from the bottom of the table rather than those of similar or higher ranking as she is more likely to win

To generate NACH and **approach behaviour**:
- ensure success by setting achievable process and performance goals
- raise confidence by giving positive reinforcement
- highlight successful role models who have comparable characteristics
- credit internal reasons, e.g. ability, for success

Avoidance behaviour arises due to a lack of self-confidence, high anxiety, learned helplessness and attributing failure internally, e.g. to low ability.

> **Tip** Short questions at the beginning of the paper often ask for the characteristics of NACH and NAF performers. Don't make the mistake of linking extrovert personalities with NACH performers — there are many NACH introverts.

Arousal

> **What the examiner will expect you to be able to do**
> - Explain and give examples for each of the three theories of arousal: drive reduction, inverted U and catastrophe theories. Draw the curves correctly and label the axes.
> - Describe adaptations to the inverted U theory and give examples (this is a common question).
> - Discuss the ZOF and how it compares with the inverted U theory, and give examples.
> - Discuss the characteristics of the ZOF, and explain what is required to enter a peak flow state. Refer to both cognitive and somatic arousal.

Arousal is the level of somatic or cognitive **stimulation** that gets us ready to perform ('**somatic**' refers to the body; '**cognitive**' refers to the mind). Being aroused to the correct level and being motivated is important in sport.

Drive reduction theory

This theory highlights the importance of maintaining motivation levels. If performers lose their drive or motivation, it has negative effects on their desire to lead an active lifestyle. They may become disaffected and sedentary.

- Performers have an initial drive or motivation to learn a new skill.
- Their drive means they will practise the skill until it is mastered/grooved.
- Success lowers their motivation levels.
- They no longer practise the skill, and may discontinue participation.
- A new goal must be presented in order to renew their drive.

For example, a youngster is determined to learn to ride his bike without stabilisers, so he practises frequently. Once he can ride the bike properly, he loses interest and no longer practises. He requires a new challenge, such as negotiating ramps, to provide further motivation and drive.

Drive theory

- As arousal increases so does performance quality, linearly.
- At high arousal the performer reverts to his/her dominant response. This is a well-learned skill that the performer uses when under immense competitive pressure.
- If the performer is in the autonomous phase of learning, or is using a gross or simple skill, the dominant response is likely to be correct.
- If the performer is in the associative phase of learning, he/she will not be able to cope with the high level of arousal and therefore the dominant response is likely to be incorrect.
- If the skill being performed is a fine or complex skill, the dominant response is likely to be incorrect.
- Inexperienced performers should participate at lower levels of arousal.
- This theory does not account for elite performers deteriorating under immense competitive pressure.

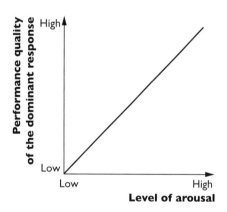

Inverted U theory

This is a more practical theory, which suggests that as arousal increases, so does performance quality, up to an optimum point at moderate arousal. Performance quality then decreases as a result of over-arousal. Under- and over-arousal are equally detrimental to performance. However, the theory does not account for the dramatic decrease in performance seen by some elite performers once they have exceeded their optimum level of arousal.

Performers who are **under-aroused** are not stimulated enough to perform. Their attentional field will be too broad, so although they are focusing on several cues around them, they miss the correct environmental cues as they are not concentrating well enough. This may lead to information overload.

At **moderate arousal**, selective attention is fully operational. The performer filters the relevant cues from the irrelevant, and concentrates completely on the specific environmental cues required to perform

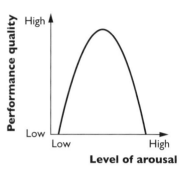

Performers who are **over-aroused** may be in a highly agitated state, experiencing 'hypervigilance' or panic. Their attentional field is narrowed, causing them again to miss the correct environmental cues. .

Modifications to the inverted U theory

Some performers operate best at high levels of arousal, while others can tolerate only low levels. Some skills require higher levels of arousal for best performance.

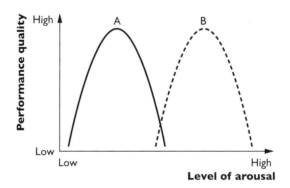

Curve A shows optimum performance occurring at lower levels of arousal. This would apply under the following circumstances:
- the performer is a novice
- fine skills are required, needing a high level of precision and control
- complex skills involving several decisions are required
- the performer is introverted and has a high resting level of adrenaline

Curve B shows optimum performance occurring at higher levels of arousal. This applies when:
- the performer is advanced
- gross skills are required — precision and control are not needed
- simple skills involving few decisions are required
- the performer is extrovert — he/she has a low resting level of adrenaline and strives for 'exciting' situations

Catastrophe theory

This theory accounts for the sudden drop in performance that can occur when optimum arousal is exceeded.

Catastrophe theory is multidimensional. It considers the effects of both cognitive and somatic anxiety. As arousal increases so does performance quality up to an optimum point at moderate arousal, as shown by the inverted U theory. However, there is then a dramatic decrease in performance as a result of high cognitive anxiety combined with high somatic anxiety. The body and the mind become over-aroused, causing an immediate decline in performance.

Techniques such as deep breathing exercises and progressive muscle relaxation can reverse the effects of over-arousal. The performer can then continue, provided a level of relaxation below the point of catastrophe has been reached.

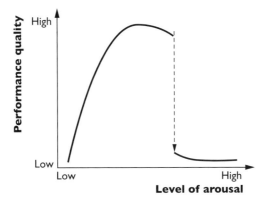

Peak flow experience

Peak flow describes the positive psychological state of performers when:

- the level of challenge they are presented with matches their skill level
- they have a clear goal
- they have the correct attentional style
- they have a positive attitude before and during the performance
- they have control of their arousal levels

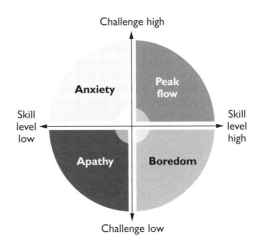

If a performer is presented with a challenge that is perceived as too great, it will result in anxiety — for instance, a novice skier attempting a black piste will undoubtedly feel nervous. If the task is too easy, the performer will become bored. For example a club-level high jumper would find it monotonous to be taught the basics with class-mates at school. Equally, a low-skilled performer presented with an easy task will take an apathetic view. To achieve peak flow, performers should be given a task that is realistic yet challenges them at an appropriate level. They then enter a rewarding psychological and physical state, known as '**the zone**'.

Hanin's zone of optimal functioning (ZOF)

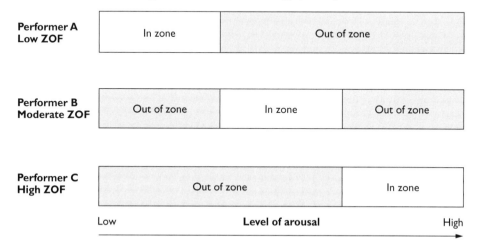

The zone is a mental state that autonomous performers experience when everything is 'perfect'. Characteristics of the zone include:
- performing at optimum arousal levels
- feeling completely calm
- complete attentional control — fully concentrated on the task with the correct attentional style
- performing on 'autopilot' — some performers have no memory of it
- feeling completely confident that success is inevitable
- performing smoothly and efficiently

Hanin suggests that optimum performance is reached during a band or zone, not at a point as described by inverted U theory. Performer A enters the zone, achieving best performance, at low levels of arousal. This could be a cognitive performer or some-one performing a fine skill such as a darts throw. Performer B is in the zone at moder-ate levels of arousal. This could be an associative performer or someone performing a skill that requires a certain level of precision such as a tennis serve. Performer C enters the zone at high levels of arousal. This relates to autonomous performers, as they are used to performing in competitive circumstances, which generate high levels of arousal. Gross skills such as a rugby tackle also need high levels of arousal and would therefore be in this band.

Controlling anxiety

What the examiner will expect you to be able to do
- Distinguish between cognitive and somatic anxiety.
- Discuss causes of anxiety and ways to eliminate them (be aware of some strong links with controlling aggression).
- Explain the difference between state and trait anxiety.
- Describe and critically evaluate the anxiety tests.
- Describe Easterbrook and Nideffer's models and apply clear examples.
- Describe the types of goals and the SMARTER principle and give examples of all types of goal.
- Explain why process/performance goals are as important as 'winning' goals.
- Discuss why goal setting is important in mental preparation and for developing confidence, concentration and emotional control. Refer to goal setting in answers on these subjects and others such as achievement motivation.

Anxiety affects performance negatively. Anxiety is caused by performers' *perception* that their ability is not good enough. They may have the necessary skills and ability to perform well and succeed but if they perceive that they don't, they begin to worry, lose focus and experience negative thoughts, which will affect performance.

Anxiety and its causes

Anxiety can be categorised as follow:
- **Trait anxiety** is where the performer is naturally anxious in all situations — his or her personality is innate, stable and enduring.
- **State anxiety** — the performer is anxious only in certain situations, often caused by negative past experiences. It is a temporary feeling but it is equally detrimental to performance. It is often seen in high-pressure situations such as taking a penalty.

The causes of anxiety include:
- task importance, e.g. playing in a final
- losing, or fear of failing
- perceived inaccuracy of an official's decisions
- being fouled
- injury, or fear of being injured
- lack of self-confidence or efficacy
- audience effects, e.g. an abusive crowd
- evaluation apprehension

Anxiety shows itself in two ways:

- **Cognitive anxiety** — mental symptoms of anxiety, e.g. worrying, irrational thoughts and confusion. Learned helplessness may occur.
- **Somatic anxiety** — physiological symptoms of anxiety, e.g. increased heart rate, blood pressure, sweat levels and muscle tension.

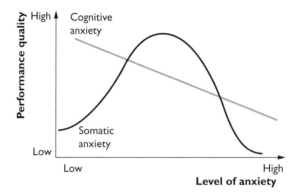

Often, both types of anxiety occur together in sport. To achieve maximal perform-ance, the athlete needs to experience low levels of cognitive anxiety and not worry about performing. As described in the inverted U theory, performers should have moderate levels of somatic anxiety as this produces the best performance. Low levels mean the performer is not stimulated enough; high levels mean excessive amounts of adrenaline in the body, increasing the likelihood of somatic symptoms occurring and reducing performance.

Measuring anxiety

Anxiety can be measured in the same manner as personality, using observation, questionnaires and physiological methods such as heart-rate monitors and measur-ing sweat. The same limitations apply and anxiety can increase when the performer knows he or she is being tested.

Self-report questionnaires are often used to measure anxiety. Martens' **sport competition anxiety test (SCAT)** was devised specifically to measure anxiety in sporting situations. Performers answer statements rating their level of anxiety. Coaches and psychologists can then evaluate which performers need help with man-aging anxiety.

The **state–trait anxiety inventory (STAI)** is a 40-question test that distinguishes between specific state and trait anxiety. Performers score themselves on a scale of 1–4 in each question, measuring feelings of nervousness, worry, apprehension, ten-sion based on the performer's current feelings (state) and general feelings (trait). The **competitive state anxiety inventory-2 (CSAI-2)** was developed to measure cog-nitive and somatic anxiety and self-confidence in competitive situations. Performers rate themselves on a 4-point scale about their feelings at that moment in response to

27 statements. Usually the inventory is given out on more than one occasion leading up to an event — for example, the week before, the day before, an hour before — as this will indicate the level, type and timing of the anxiety experienced. This method is limited as it is a self-report questionnaire — the performer may not answer truthfully.

Managing anxiety

Many performers experience high levels of anxiety when participating. If they fail to manage their anxiety, they may well refrain from participating. Performers should be taught a range of strategies that enable them to manage their anxiety levels.

Cognitive strategies
- **Mental rehearsal** — go over the performance in your mind, e.g. a triple jumper visualises all the sub-routines without moving.
- **Imagery** — recall a successful previous performance, use all the senses including kinaesthesis to recreate the feeling of success, e.g. a tennis player remembers how the serve felt when she hit an ace.
- **Positive self-talk** — remind yourself verbally of the key points of the movement and tell yourself that you can achieve, e.g. a rugby league player taking a conversion talks himself through the run-up, contact and follow-through, telling himself he can take the points. He may keep repeating a **mantra**.
- **Negative-thought stopping** — often used with the above, e.g. a tennis player whose serve is letting her down replaces the thought 'I can't hit one in' with 'I can and I will hit the next one in'.
- **Rational or positive thinking** — as a performer you experience anxiety when you *perceive* that you are not good enough. You should look at the task subjectively and think logically that you can and will be successful.
- **Selective attention** — focus on the relevant environmental stimuli and disregard the irrelevant, e.g. a footballer taking a penalty focuses on the ball and goal, not the crowd.

Somatic strategies
- **Progressive muscular relaxation** — concentrate on each muscle group in turn. By tensing, holding then relaxing each group, you begin to relax.
- **Biofeedback** — physiological data are generated using equipment such as heart-rate monitors while you undertake various tasks. The data show which approach is best for you. This is an effective but time-consuming strategy. Using equipment during performance can be distracting and increase anxiety levels.
- **Deep breathing** — by controlling and concentrating on the rate and depth of breathing, you becomes less distracted, allowing yourself to focus on the task.
- **Centring** — this is used alongside controlled breathing and is useful during breaks in performance, e.g. time-outs or the end of a tennis set. Concentrate fully on your body (often the centre, i.e. your belly-button region) and breathe in. As you breathe out, chant a word or phrase describing how you wish to perform (you are strong, focused, calm etc.). This maintains focus on yourself and negative thoughts are disregarded.

Coaches' strategies
- Set performance and process goals, not product goals.
- Ensure success by setting easy targets.
- Ensure skills are over-learned.
- Raise self-efficacy.
- Give positive reinforcement.
- Remind the performer of successful past experiences.
- Encourage performers to attribute success internally.

Attentional control

During performance athletes concentrate on a range of environmental cues. If they can quickly identify and focus on the essential elements, their performance will improve. They will avoid distraction, so reducing the risk of information overload. In addition, reaction time will improve. They also increase the likelihood of entering the ZOF.

Cue utilisation
Easterbrook's cue utilisation hypothesis links a performer's ability to sustain focus on the correct cues in the environment with the level of arousal he or she is experiencing. At low levels of arousal, the performer is not stimulated enough and takes in a large number of environmental cues. He or she is unable to distinguish what the relevant cues are and can become confused, reducing performance level. At high levels of arousal, the performer takes in a small number of cues because he or she is excessively stimulated and may begin to panic. The correct cues are missed, again reducing performance level. At moderate levels of arousal, the performer is able to filter out the irrelevant cues and focus only on the cues required. The performer completes the task to the highest level. Easterbrook therefore supports the inverted U theory of arousal, which also suggests that performance is best at moderate levels of arousal.

Nideffer suggested that different sporting activities require different types of attentional control. For example, invasion games often require a broad attentional focus, whereas net or wall games may need a narrower style. Performers are required to apply a variety of styles, with the best athletes being able to switch from one to another readily. There are two **dimensions of focus**:
- **Broad–narrow** — the number of cues being focused on: 'broad' is many; 'narrow' is one or two.
- **Internal–external** — the location of the focus: 'internal' focuses on the thoughts and feelings of the performer herself; 'external' deals with environmental cues.

Four **attentional styles** arise from this:
- **Broad–internal** — the focus is on many cues concerning the performer himself, e.g. a footballer planning team strategies or the next set piece.
- **Narrow–internal** — the focus is on one or two cues concerning the performer himself; often used to calm nerves, e.g. a swimmer mentally rehearsing the starter signal and his subsequent dive into the pool.

- **Broad–external** — the focus is on many cues in the environment, e.g. a centre player in netball focusing on several team mates prior to making a pass.
- **Narrow–external** — the focus is on one or two cues in the environment, e.g. a basketballer focusing on the net during a free throw.

Goal setting

Psychological research has shown that setting goals has a positive effect on performance. Generally, performers who set goals are more committed, maintain participation and are more task-persistent. The benefits of setting goals include:

- giving the performer an aim or focus
- increasing motivation when the goal is accomplished
- increasing confidence levels
- controlling arousal/anxiety levels
- focusing efforts in training and game situations

Types of goals

- **Process goals** — relatively short-term goals set to improve technique, e.g. an ice dancer aims to improve her toe loop technique.
- **Performance goals** — intermediate goals often set against yourself to improve performance from last time, e.g. to gain a higher mark than in the previous competition.
- **Product goals** — long-term goals reached after extensive work. These are often set against others and are based on the outcome, e.g. to win the county ice-dance championships.

Short-term and intermediate goals are motivational as they are often achieved quickly. They build confidence as the performer receives feedback and therefore continues to strive towards more advanced goals. Long-term goals provide the performer with a final aim. When setting goals, it is important that the coach and performer do not focus solely on the outcome of winning, as this increases the likelihood of failure, causing anxiety for the performer and lowering motivation. Shorter process and performance goals should be set. When running a marathon, for instance, instead of setting the unrealistic product goal of winning, the athlete should aim to achieve a personal best (PB) time.

Principles of goal setting

When setting goals the SMARTER principle should be followed:

	Explanation	Example
Specific	The goal must be precise	Reach level 10.5 on the multi-stage fitness test
Measurable	The goal must be quantifiable	Make ten tackles in the next half
Agreed	The goal must be concurred by the performer and the coach so they share responsibility	You and your coach decide to reduce your 400 m time by 2 s

	Explanation	Example
Realistic	It must be within the performer's reach	Aim to run 10 km in under 55 min
Time-phased	A set period must be stated	Perform a PB time in the 100 m freestyle by the end of next month
Exciting	The goal has to be motivational	Learn to do a somersault on the trampoline by next week
Recorded	The progress has to be written down	The coach will document the height of every high jump you make

Attitudes

What the examiner will expect you to be able to do
- Describe the three components of an attitude and how they are formed, with clear examples.
- Explain prejudice and give examples.
- Describe cognitive dissonance and persuasive communication.

An attitude describes an individual's predisposition to believe, feel and act towards an attitude object. Attitude objects are the focus of an attitude and can include people, places, situations and items. An individual's attitude plays an important role in the development of an active lifestyle, particularly for young people. If they hold a positive attitude towards physical activity, they are more likely to participate. However, a negative attitude may lead to a sedentary lifestyle and the possibility of developing diseases related to being inactive. Attitudes are usually deep rooted but can be changed. It is imperative that teachers and coaches generate positive attitudes to encourage and maintain participation and encourage healthier lifestyle choices.

Origins of attitudes

Attitudes can be positive or negative. They develop through experiences rather than being innate and often begin to form at an early age. They develop for a number of reasons.

Past experiences
Winning matches or titles, for example, is an enjoyable experience that can lead to the development of a positive attitude. The individual then develops a perception of his or her own ability as high, which increases confidence and can help to build a positive attitude towards active lifestyle pastimes. A bad experience, such as losing or injury, can have the opposite effect. The performer may develop low self-confidence and a perception of their own ability as low. This may lead to a negative attitude towards physical activity as a whole, and to learned helplessness.

Socialisation

This describes how individuals want to fit in with the **cultural norms** surrounding them. This is particularly important with school-age children. If it is the norm for your friendship group or family to participate in physical activity regularly, then you will conform and have a positive attitude towards sport. If, for example, they all play for a team or attend the gym regularly, you do the same because you don't want to feel left out. However, if it is the norm for your peers and family not to participate, and they hold negative attitudes, you will adopt these to be consistent with those around you. A sedentary lifestyle may result.

Social learning

This involves imitating the attitudes of significant others such as parents, teachers and peers. If your parents and friends have a positive attitude towards physical activity, it is likely that you will copy them, especially if you are reinforced or praised for doing so. Conversely, if they hold negative attitudes and your parents and friends abstain from participating, it is likely that you will do the same.

Media

High-profile role models in the media often display positive attitudes and, as we respect them, we are likely to adopt their positive attitudes towards being active.

Prejudice

Prejudice is a biased judgement made before all the relevant facts have been gathered. It is often based on race, gender, age, physical ability, sexual orientation or negative attitudes towards officials or the police. It is detrimental to sport. It can reduce participation in certain groups — for instance, a female footballer, jeered at by a group of male peers on the grounds that 'girls can't play football', may stop participating.

Prejudice may develop due to:
- **Social learning and/or socialisation** — you learn prejudice from significant others and also to fit in with the norm, e.g. if your family and friends shout racist abuse at a player, you may copy them to be part of the group.
- **Past experience** — one negative past experience, e.g. a referee giving away a debatable penalty against your team, leads you to become prejudiced towards all officials.
- **Media hype** — television and newspapers regularly hype up matches, particularly local derbies or those where the teams are associated with religious groups, e.g. Celtic versus Rangers. This may increase prejudice.

The components of attitudes

The **triadic model** suggests that an attitude is made up of three components:
- **Cognitive**: beliefs or thoughts — e.g. 'I believe that attending the gym helps me to lead a balanced, active and healthy lifestyle.'
- **Affective**: emotions and feelings — e.g. 'I enjoy attending the various classes at the gym and feel energised afterwards.'

- **Behavioural**: actions and responses — e.g. 'I attend the gym five times each week.'

However, attitudes are inconsistent. A performer may believe that attending the gym is good for him or her and enjoy it but may not attend due to lack of time or motivation. Beliefs don't always correspond with behaviour and therefore attitudes are poor predictors of behaviour.

Changing attitudes and prejudice

It is important to be able to change the negative attitude of people who do not participate in physical activity and lead an inactive lifestyle, or who show prejudiced behaviour.

Some strategies include:
- **persuasive communication**, particularly by significant others
- ensuring **positive, successful experiences**
- **praising positive attitudes** and non-prejudicial behaviour
- **punishing prejudice**, e.g. substitution or bans
- **using positive role models** in the media to highlight positive attitudes towards activity or non-prejudicial behaviour
- **merging groups** so that individuals work together across gender, age etc.
- **generating cognitive dissonance**

Cognitive dissonance

When an individual's attitude components all match, whether positively or negatively, they are in a state of **cognitive consonance**. Their beliefs, feelings and actions are in harmony and the individual's attitude will be stable. One way to change an attitude is to create **cognitive dissonance**. Dissonance is caused by generating unease in the individual. This can be done by changing one of more of the negative attitude components into a positive, thus causing the individual to question their attitude. This may lead an inactive individual into a balanced and healthier lifestyle.

	Negative attitude	Change by
Cognitive	I think that going to the gym is a waste of time	Education, preferably by a significant other. Explain that attending the gym can make you healthy. It creates muscle tone, improves appearance and reduces the risk of disease
Affective	I hate going to the gym	A positive, varied experience. Make it fun/enjoyable. Ensure that the individual is successful
Behavioural	I don't go to the gym	Persuasive communication, preferably by a specialist. Praise the individual to reinforce their behaviour so they continue to participate

Tip Questions on changing attitudes are common, so revise cognitive dissonance and persuasive communication thoroughly.

Aggression

What the examiner will expect you to be able to do
- Give definitions and clear examples of the types of aggression and assertion; this is a grey area.
- Discuss the nature versus nurture debate on aggression and describe the theories of aggression.
- Describe strategies to reduce aggression and give a range of answers.

Hostile aggression is when an individual purposefully harms or injures an opponent for no reason other than to inflict pain. It is outside the rules and anger is shown, for instance when a rugby league player punches his opponent as he gets up to play the ball.

Instrumental aggression is also when an individual purposefully harms or injures an opponent, however here the aim is *not* to harm or injure but to gain an advantage over the opposition. Anger is not involved. An example is a hockey defender hitting the ankle of a quick, agile forward with her stick. The intent is to slow her down and therefore gain an advantage, rather than to make her suffer.

Assertion is often confused with aggression. This is when an individual plays hard but within the rules, perhaps using more effort than usual. There is no intention to harm the opposition. For instance, a strong, quick bowl at the batter in rounders and a crunching but fair tackle in rugby union are both assertive play.

Aggression should be channelled, which means all the performer's effort and energy is redirected into positive, assertive play rather than negative aggressive reactions. There are many causes of aggression including:
- losing
- playing badly
- team-mates not trying
- unfair officials' decisions
- provocation by an opponent or the crowd
- contact sport, e.g. ice hockey, Gaelic football

Theories of aggression

Instinct theory
As humans, we have an inherited predisposition to be aggressive. We have a natural tendency to defend ourselves and in sport, our territory. Instinct theorists believe that aggression builds up within us inevitably and we require a positive outlet, such as sporting activity, to release it. This is known as **catharsis**. For example, after a hard week at work you release your aggression by playing football and making several aggressive tackles.

This theory has the following drawbacks:
- It does not consider the effect of environment or social learning on aggression.
- Individuals often experience increased aggression during sporting competition rather than it having a cathartic effect.
- Different societal groups exhibit varying levels of aggressive tendencies, with some showing none at all. The instinct approach suggests that we are all genetically pre-determined to behave aggressively.

Frustration–aggression hypothesis

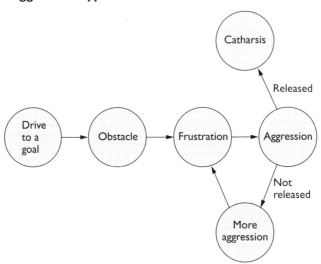

When a performer has a drive to achieve a goal but is prevented from doing so, he/she experiences frustration. Frustration always leads to an aggressive response. For example, a basketball player dribbling towards the basket is fouled and his goal is blocked. He feels frustrated and strikes an opposition player. This has a cathartic effect, reducing frustration and aggression. If the player is then punished by the officials, he experiences even more frustration.

This theory does not account for:
- Performers who experience frustration and aggression even when goals have not been blocked.
- Performers who have their goals blocked and experience frustration but do not react aggressively.

Aggressive cue hypothesis
Berkowitz updated the frustration–aggression hypothesis. When a performer's goal is blocked, her arousal levels increase and she experiences frustration. This leads to her being *ready* for an aggressive act, rather than aggression being inevitable. An aggressive act will only happen if learned cues or triggers are present. For example, aggressive objects such as bats and clubs or aggressive contact sports such as rugby and ice hockey are more likely to produce aggressive responses.

Social learning theory

This opposes the trait approach to aggression and is based on the work of **Bandura**. Aggression is learned by watching and copying the behaviour of significant others. If an aggressive act is reinforced or is successful, it is more likely to be copied. For example, a young rugby player watches his idol high-tackle an opponent. The crowd cheers and the opponent is prevented from scoring a try. As this aggressive act is reinforced and successful, the young player copies this behaviour. Performers may also become aggressive due to socialisation. For instance, a footballer observes his team-mates shouting abuse and acting aggressively towards the referee as they disagree with a penalty call. He joins in to fit in with his colleagues. Aggression is more likely to be copied if the model shares characteristics with the performer. This theory does not take into account genetic explanations as to why aggression occurs — it discounts the trait approach even though recent studies have shown that there may be an aggressive/angry gene in humans.

> **Tip** The extended question may ask you to discuss the nature versus nurture debate on aggression or simply to describe the theories of aggression. To gain the highest marks, address the topics with clear examples.

Eliminating aggression

Performers who are repeatedly subjected to aggression may feel intimidated and stressed, lose concentration and/or self-esteem or become injured. It is therefore important that undesirable aggressive acts are eliminated from sport.

Players	Coaches
Cognitive techniques • Mental rehearsal • Imagery • Visualisation • Selective attention • Negative-thought stopping • Positive self-talk Somatic techniques • Relaxation techniques • Deep breathing • Biofeedback General techniques • Count to 10 • Walk away • Mantra • Displace aggressive feelings by playing hard, e.g. kicking the ball harder	Praise non-aggressive acts Highlight non-aggressive role models Punish aggression, e.g. substitution/fines Use peer pressure to remind one another that aggression is unacceptable Set process and performance goals rather than product goals Ensure their own behaviour is not aggressive Give the performer responsibility within the team

> **Tip** When asked for strategies to reduce aggression, give a range of answers as some will appear on the same point on the mark scheme and you will only receive credit once.

Confidence

What the examiner will expect you to be able to do
- Describe the four key components of Bandura's model with clear examples and explain the links with achievement motivation and attribution theory.
- Explain the positive *and* negative effects of an audience.
- Explain the links with selective attention and the peak flow experience.
- Describe and apply the distraction conflict theory and the home-field advantage

A performer's natural, innate confidence is called **trait sports confidence**. For instance, a performer may be generally confident and will show this in all situations. However, some performers are confident only in specific tasks, sports or situations. This is known as **state sports confidence** or **self-efficacy** and is linked to positive past experiences. For example, a performer may be confident that he will score a conversion because he has done so many times before.

Bandura's self-efficacy theory

Self-efficacy describes the amount of confidence a performer has in a particular sporting situation. It is specific rather than general and varies with circumstance. Bandura suggested that four factors influence the level of self-efficacy shown by a performer. By addressing these factors, coaches and teachers can raise performers' self-efficacy, resulting in a more positive and successful performance. Often, individuals lead a sedentary lifestyle because they have low confidence in their sporting ability and low self-esteem. By raising their efficacy levels in one area, coaches may increase a performer's self-esteem and belief in their ability to master other tasks. This may lead to higher participation levels and a more active lifestyle.

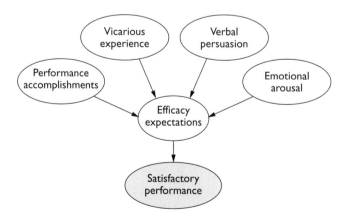

For example, a young gymnast is anxious when asked to perform on a full-height beam. To increase her self-efficacy, the coach should use the four factors described below.

- **Performance accomplishments**: remind her of past successes in similar situations — that she was brilliant on the lower beam and didn't fall off; the beam is the same width, so she is equally unlikely to fall.
- **Vicarious experiences**: use a role model who shares her characteristics (ability, gender, age etc.) to show what she can achieve — ask a gymnast of similar age and standard to perform on the beam; the young gymnast will say, 'If she can do it, so can I'.
- **Verbal persuasion**: encourage her and tell her that she can succeed. Enhance this by using significant others — the coach and friends of the gymnast must persuade her that they believe she can perform well on the beam.
- **Emotional arousal**: show her how to control arousal levels using cognitive and somatic strategies. Psychological and physiological symptoms of over-arousal (increased heart rate, sweating etc.) can reduce self-efficacy as she perceives that she cannot achieve her goal. The coach must tell her to rehearse, in her mind, the moves on the beam before mounting, so that she can focus and lower her arousal levels.

Social facilitation and inhibition

Some people enjoy performing with an audience and their performance improves. This is known as **social facilitation**. It may result in performers being motivated to participate and so lead an active lifestyle. Others dislike performing with an audience, and their performance worsens when being observed. This is known as **social inhibition**. Many such performers lose motivation because they cannot deal with the pressure. They may decide to avoid sporting situations altogether and lead a sedentary lifestyle.

> **Tip** To understand social facilitation fully you need to have a good knowledge of arousal, so go back over your notes. Bring arousal into your answers if it is relevant, particularly in the extended-answer questions.

Passive and interactive others

Zajonc suggested that four types of 'others' may be present during performance.

'Passive others' do not interact with the performer but have an effect simply by being present:

- the **audience** — does not speak but watches, e.g. silent observers during a tee-off in golf, or a scout who arrives to observe a performance. Their mere presence can make you anxious and affect your game.
- **co-actors** — perform the same task at the same time but do not compete against you, e.g. the sight of another cyclist in front that makes you speed up to overtake. Although you win nothing by doing so, their presence has made you cycle faster.

'Interactive others' communicate directly with the performer:
- **competitive co-actors** — the opposition, e.g. other swimmers in direct rivalry with the performer during a race.
- **supporters** — the crowd, e.g. spectators at a rugby match who cheer and applaud but may also shout abuse at performers. They may give you the motivation to improve.

Even when others present are passive, the main effect on the performer is increased arousal levels. The presence of an audience has the same varied effects on performance as arousal, as illustrated by the inverted U hypothesis.

Factors facilitating and inhibiting performance

Performance will be facilitated if the performer is:
- an expert used to performing in front of an audience
- performing a gross skill (large muscle group movements) that does not require precision or accuracy
- performing a simple skill, which requires limited decision making or information processing
- an extrovert who seeks social situations and has low levels of natural arousal — his/her RAS is activated only with high levels of stimulation. The presence of an audience is seen as an opportunity to 'show off' and rise to the challenge.

In the above circumstances the performer will be able to cope with the additional arousal caused by presence of the audience and the performance will improve.

Performance will be inhibited if the performer is:
- a novice who finds performing in front of an audience intimidating
- performing a fine skill (that requires precision and accuracy), which is difficult to maintain at high arousal
- performing a complex skill requiring several decisions to be made and a lot of information processing, which may not be performed successfully at high arousal
- an introvert who dislikes social situations and has high levels of natural arousal — his or her RAS is activated with low levels of stimulation. He or she finds performing in front of others demanding and this will have a detrimental effect on performance.

In the above circumstances the performer cannot cope with the extra arousal, which means the performance will deteriorate.

Zajonc based his model on Hull's drive theory. This suggests that, at high levels of arousal, performers revert to their **dominant response** — a well-learned skill that the performer will use when under immense competitive pressure. Experts will store over-learned motor programmes in their long-term memory and their dominant response is likely to be performed correctly. Therefore performance will be facilitated. If the response is gross or simple, or is performed by an extrovert, it will be facilitated.

Novices, however, have not yet grooved their responses. By being under competitive pressure and in the presence of an audience, their performance will be inhibited. A fine or complex skill response or an introverted performer will be inhibited.

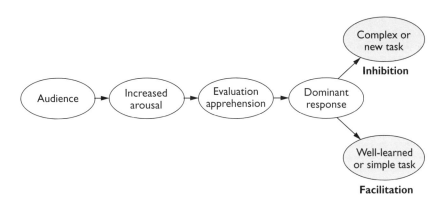

Evaluation apprehension

This is the **fear of being judged**. It causes the performer to revert to the dominant response. If a performer *perceives* that he or she is being judged, it will have an effect on the performance. Other factors that can cause evaluation apprehension include:

- a knowledgeable audience, e.g. the presence of a scout
- the presence of significant others such as parents or peers — positive and negative effects are seen depending on the task and performers, as described above
- whether an audience is supportive or abusive, which will facilitate or inhibit performance
- naturally high trait anxiety, which will make a performer inhibited by an audience
- low self-efficacy, which will make a performer doubt his or her ability and cause inhibition

Home-field advantage

Performance is usually better when playing at home due to having a large number of supporters present, not having to travel and being familiar with the venue. This keeps uncertainty and therefore arousal levels low. If the audience is close to the playing area, home-field advantage is even more important — for example, in basketball. However, during the later stages of a competition, the pressure may be high when playing at home owing to the crowd's expectations of winning, therefore causing inhibition.

Baron's distraction conflict theory

This suggests that during performance we pay attention to the task in hand but we may also pay attention to 'distracters'. These could come from external sources such as the crowd or internal sources such as negative thoughts. Paying attention to both the task and the distracters causes a psychological conflict, which increases arousal. This leads to either social facilitation or inhibition, depending on the type of task and the ability level of the performer. For example, a footballer taking a penalty is concentrating on the task — the ball and goal. Crowd members behind the goal cause a distraction by shouting at the player, which diverts some of his attention away from the task. This causes psychological conflict and arousal levels increase. If he is an expert, it is likely that his performance will be facilitated and he will score. If he is a

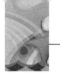

cognitive performer, he will be unable to deal with the increased arousal caused by the crowd. Therefore his performance may be inhibited and he may miss.

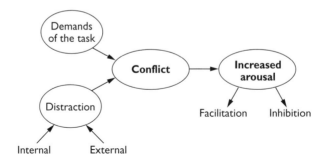

Strategies to combat social inhibition

- Familiarisation training: allow an audience to watch you training, or play crowd noise during training.
- Increase self-efficacy (see Bandura's model).
- Practise skills until they are grooved.
- Selective attention: block out the crowd and concentrate on the relevant stimuli such as the ball or the opposition.

Use other cognitive strategies such as:
- mental rehearsal
- imagery
- positive self-talk
- negative-thought stopping

In addition the coach could:
- decrease the importance of the task
- support the performer by offering encouragement, positive reinforcement and praise

Attribution theory

What the examiner will expect you to be able to do
- Apply Weiner's model to sporting situations.
- Define the key terms relating to Weiner's model, including mastery orientation, learned helplessness, self-serving bias and attributional retraining.
- Explain the links with achievement motivation.
- Explain how coaches can reduce learned helplessness and promote mastery orientation in performers to create a healthy lifestyle.

Attribution theory describes how individuals explain their behaviour. In a sporting context, performers use attributions to offer reasons when they win or lose.

Weiner's attribution model

Locus of causality

	Internal	External
Stable	**Ability**	**Task difficulty**
Unstable	**Effort**	**Luck**

(Vertical axis label: Locus of stability)

Weiner suggested that four key attributions lie on two dimensions:

The **locus of causality** describes where the performer places the reason for winning or losing:
- **internal** — within the performer's control, e.g. the amount of natural ability possessed or the amount of effort put into training
- **external** — out of the performer's control and determined by the environment, e.g. task difficulty (the level of opposition faced) or luck (decisions made by officials or environmental factors such as an unlucky ball bounce)

The **stability dimension** describes how fixed the attributions are:
- **stable** — the reason is relatively permanent, e.g. the ability (internal, stable) of the performer remains the same over a long period of time, as does the task difficulty (e.g. ability of the opposition — external, stable)
- **unstable** or changeable — this change could be from week to week or even within minutes, e.g. the effort (internal, unstable) shown to chase down a ball may be higher when winning at the beginning of the match than towards the end of the same match when losing. Luck (external, unstable) is also changeable, e.g. the officials

Mastery orientation

Mastery-orientated performers attribute success to internal reasons such as 'We were the better team', or 'We put more effort into training.' Attributing in this way raises the self-efficacy of performers, who will feel content and able to repeat their success in the future. Because their confidence is high, they may be motivated to continue participating. They show the characteristics of NACH performers and will not give up if they do not succeed. They are persistent. When mastery-orientated performers fail, they attribute this to external factors such as task difficulty or luck — for instance, the referee gave the 50/50 offside call to the opposition. They feel that failure can be overcome if they try harder. Not all performers show this level of persistence and some develop learned helplessness.

Learned helplessness

Learned helplessness develops when performers attribute failure internally to stable reasons, for instance 'I lost the swimming race because I simply haven't got the ability'. They believe that no matter what they do they are destined to fail and they therefore lack persistence. Learned helplessness can be general and relate to all sports ('I cannot play any sport') or specific, relating to one skill ('I can't take penalty flicks in hockey as I will miss') or a single sport ('I can't play badminton'). It usually occurs when performers have low self-confidence due to past failings; they withdraw and stop participating. It may also be due to unrealistic goals set by a coach. Performers with learned helplessness share similar characteristics to NAF performers, and if their attributions remain unchanged, they will probably lead a sedentary lifestyle because of their low sporting self-esteem.

To reduce the effects of learned helplessness, performers should change their negative attributions into positive ones. This is called **attribution retraining**. Performers and coaches alike should always attribute the reasons for winning internally (to ability and effort) rather than externally (e.g. luck). Failure should be attributed externally rather than internally. This is known as **self-serving bias**. Attributing success internally raises self-efficacy and esteem and increases the likelihood of an individual continuing to participate, sustaining an active lifestyle.

Apart from attribution retraining, to build a mastery-orientated approach coaches should:
- set realistic process and/or performance goals
- raise self-efficacy using Bandura's model
- highlight previous quality performances
- give positive reinforcement and encouragement

Group success

What the examiner will expect you to be able to do
- Define the term 'group'.
- Define the various aspects of Steiner's model.
- Account for the factors relating to the formation of a group and its cohesion.
- Discuss task and social cohesion and give clear examples to support your answers.

Group dynamics is the study of groups and group members. It includes how groups operate, for instance group expectations or norms, the relationships within the group, and how effectively groups interact with each other. A group is two or more people who:

- interact with each other, i.e. communicate
- share a common goal, i.e. have the same aim
- have mutual awareness, i.e. influence and depend on each other

Tuckman suggested that, in order to become a group rather than a collection of individuals, members go through four key stages: forming, storming, norming and performing.

1 Forming	2 Storming
• Working out if he/she belongs in the group • Learning about other members/coaches • Developing social relationships • Working out the goal • Relying on coach to bring the group closer Example: during your first training sessions you decide that you want to be part of the hockey team because they seem to share your passion to win. You begin to socialise with other team members	• Infighting and conflict • Teams often fold • Confrontation with the leaders • Members actively challenge for their role/position • Self-preservation is important Example: both you and another team member want to be goalkeeper, which causes rivalry between you. Or you may believe that the captain is not a strong enough leader and that you could do a better job
3 Norming	**4 Performing**
• Conflicts resolved • Group cohesion develops as members become unified • Norms are set • Members cooperate to achieve potential • Motivation and success levels rise Example: you decide that your team-mate is an effective goalkeeper and that you can use your skills in an out-field position to give the team an excellent defence. You respect the captain and are aware of his/her qualities	• Group stabilised • Fully focused on achieving group success • Motivation and enjoyment is high • Respect for other members and leaders is high Example: your team plays regularly and members praise each other for team success, which is increasing now you are a unit

Steiner's model of group performance

actual productivity = potential productivity − losses due to faulty processes

Actual productivity is a team's level of achievement on a specific task, for instance a netball team reaching the semi-final of a cup competition.

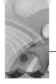

Potential productivity is the team's best possible level of achievement when it is cohesive, for instance the netball team winning the cup competition.

Losses due to faulty processes are the *coordination* and *motivation* problems the team faces, which reduce the level of cohesion and therefore lower the level of achievement, for instance the motivation levels of some team members were lower than expected and so the team didn't win the cup final.

Steiner suggested that teams face many problems that affect their productivity, including:
- coordination problems — team members fail to communicate properly with each other, resulting in poor timing or set plays breaking down
- lack of understanding of members' roles in the team
- lack of understanding of tactics or strategies set by the coach
- the Ringelmann effect
- motivation losses, such as team members withdrawing effort when training and/ or competing
- social loafing

The **Ringelmann effect** and **social loafing** are faulty processes that have a detrimental effect on the cohesiveness and attainment of a team. Long-term effects include performers withdrawing from and/or avoiding sporting activity altogether.

The Ringelmann effect was suggested after a tug-of-war experiment showed that eight participants failed to pull eight times as hard as a single participant. Ringelmann's study found that as the number of people in the group increases, the level of performance of individuals in the group decreases. For example, a rugby union player performs much better when playing in a seven-a-side tournament than when playing in a full fifteen-a-side game. It was suggested that the reduction in performance in the tug-of-war was due to lack of coordination, that is, they were not all pulling on the rope in unison. However, follow-up studies showed that the reduced performance may have been due to *lower motivation* rather than loss of coordination.

Social loafing is when performers lower the effort they contribute to the team. This happens when performers believe they are not valued as members of the group and that their input is going unnoticed, so they stop trying. If the coach does not praise you when you feel you have played well, you will eventually give up. Other factors that may cause performers to loaf include:
- no clear role within the group, e.g. they are unsure of their position within the team
- low self-efficacy/confidence, e.g. they do not believe they are good enough
- learned helplessness
- team-mates are not trying so they do the same, e.g. a winger fails to chase a ball which goes into touch, so other players think 'Why should I bother?'
- poor leadership — the coach or captain does not encourage performers or uses weak strategies
- high levels of trait or state anxiety

- injury, e.g. a twisted ankle in training means a tennis player does not reach to return wide serves
- social inhibition due to an offensive crowd

> **Tip** Short-style questions may ask you to describe a group or team and the various aspects of Steiner's model. Learn these as they offer easy marks to pick up in the exam.

Group cohesion

A cohesive team has unity and everyone pulls together to reach their shared aim. The more cohesive a team is, the more successful it will be; and the more successful the team is, the more cohesive it becomes. Two types of cohesiveness are shown within a group. The most effective groups show *both*.

Task cohesion — group members work in unity to meet a common aim. They may not socialise away from the team and may not share views but they come together to achieve their potential in the sporting arena and can get good results. This is important in interactive sports such as football and volleyball where the team members must cooperate, work together and rely on one another's timing and coordination.

Social cohesion — this occurs when group members get along and feel attached to others. They communicate and support one another within and outside the sporting arena. This is important in more co-active sports where you perform individually but your effort contributes to a whole team performance, for instance the Davis Cup in tennis or in a swimming team.

Task and social cohesion are reasons for being attracted to the group — other members share your goal of winning and you want to join because your friends are members. Or you integrate with the group to work effectively towards your goal and to get along socially with the other members.

Carron's antecedents

Carron suggested that there are four factors or **antecedents** that affect task and social cohesion. These factors can bring a team together, making it more effective, stable and satisfied. The factors are:

- **environmental** — whether a player has a contract or scholarship; the location, age and size of the group
- **leadership** — leadership style and relationships between the leader and group members
- **personal** — level of motivation shown, how satisfied you feel within the group and shared individual characteristics, e.g. age, gender, ability etc.
- **team** — the stability of the group, common experiences in victory and defeat, and a common will to win

By raising cohesiveness within a team and reducing faulty processes such as social loafing, the coach can improve individual and whole-team performances. The more an individual feels valued by and part of a team, the more likely it is that he or she will continue to participate. Coaches can:

- highlight individual performances, e.g. give statistics on shots on target, tackles, assists etc.
- give specific roles and responsibility within the team
- develop social cohesion, e.g. team-building exercises, tours, encouraging friend-ship etc.
- praise or reward cohesive behaviour, e.g. give encouragement when members work as a team
- raise individuals' confidence
- encourage group identity, e.g. have a set kit
- provide effective leadership that matches the preferred style of the group
- select players who work well together rather than individual 'stars'
- set achievable process or performance goals rather than product team goals
- emphasise the team goal continually
- select players who are less liable to social loafing
- punish social loafing
- groove set plays or do substantial coordination practice

Tip While it is not essential to know psychologists' names, it is desirable to give them wherever possible in the exam. It shows the examiner that you have read and understood the studies relating to this unit.

Leadership

What the examiner will expect you to be able to do
- State the qualities of a good leader.
- Give clear descriptions and examples of the various leadership styles and their effectiveness.
- Describe and give examples of Fiedler's model.
- Describe and give examples of Chelladurai's model.

Effective leaders are often ambitious, have a clear vision or goal and have the ability to motivate others to achieve that goal. Leaders may be:
- charismatic
- knowledgeable and/or skilful in the sport
- good communicators
- empathetic
- confident
- flexible

Prescribed leaders are chosen from outside the group, for instance national gov-erning bodies appoint national team managers. They often bring new ideas but can cause disagreements if group members are opposed to the appointment.

Emergent leaders are selected from within the group, often being nominated by the other group members. For example, a Sunday league football team might vote the previous season's 'players' player' as the new captain. There is already a high level of respect for this person but since his or her experiences are similar to other team members', he or she may not be able to bring new strategies to help the team progress.

Leadership styles

Autocratic/task-orientated	Democratic/social-orientated	Laissez-faire
Dictatorial in style Where only interest is in ensuring the task is fulfilled Sole decision-maker Use in dangerous situations, if time is limited, with large groups, hostile groups, or cognitive performers Preferred by male performers	Where interest is in ensuring relationships are developed within the group Group members are involved in making decisions Use when plenty of time is available, with small groups, friendly groups, or advanced performers Preferred by female performers	Leader is more of a 'figurehead' than an active leader Group members make all the decisions Useful if a problem-solving approach is required Only effective with advanced performers

Fiedler's contingency model

Fiedler suggested an interactionist approach in which effective leaders match their style to the situation. One of two leadership styles should be adopted:

- **Task-orientated leaders** are concerned with achieving set goals and take a pragmatic approach. They are direct and authoritarian. This style should be used both in the most and least favourable situations.
- **Person-orientated leaders** focus on developing harmony and good relationships within the group. They are open to suggestions and take a more democratic approach. This style should be used in moderately favourable situations.

The **favourableness of the situation** dictates the leadership style that should be adopted. In **most favourable** situations, the leader is in a strong position of authority and has the respect of the group, the members have good relationships with one another and the task is clear. For example, a team that has played together for many years under the same captain and where there are good relationships may have well-rehearsed set plays. When the captain calls the play, the team members know what should happen and complete the move immediately. In this situation, a task-orientated approach works best.

In **least favourable** situations, the leader has no power or respect from the group, there may be infighting in the group and hostility towards the leader, and the task is unclear. For example, a supply teacher is asked to take a year 9 PE class. She does not know the students, the group does not show any respect and the teacher is unclear as to what activities to teach. In this situation a task-orientated approach is needed to motivate the students and ensure an activity could take place.

Task-orientated leadership should be used with cognitive performers, with large groups, when time is limited and in dangerous situations. Males prefer this style.

In **moderately favourable situations**, the leader chooses a person-orientated style, which allows other team members to contribute to the decision-making process. The leader has some power and respect, some good relationships and parts of the task are clear. For example, if two new players join a netball team, the whole team discusses which positions are best for them.

Person-orientated leadership should also be used with advanced performers, with smaller groups, when there is plenty of time and when tasks are not dangerous. Females prefer this style.

> **Tip** When describing Fiedler's model, use the correct terminology — 'task-orientated' not 'autocratic', and 'person-orientated' not 'democratic'.

Chelladurai's multi-dimensional model of leadership

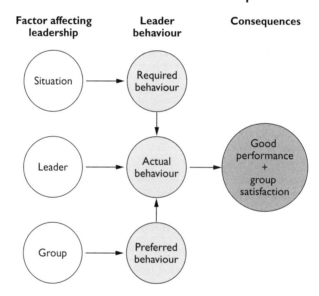

Chelladurai's model suggests that leaders must be able to adapt. They must consider three factors:

- The **situation** — e.g. the strength of the opponent or whether any danger is involved. For example, learning to trampoline is dangerous and requires an autocratic approach.
- **Themselves** — e.g. their ability, personality and preferred leadership style. For example, the leader is experienced and prefers to use an autocratic style.
- The **group** — e.g. the group's ability, the relationships within the group and with the leader. For example, the group comprises cognitive performers and therefore needs to be given direct instructions about how to perform moves on the trampoline bed.

Leadership style is also affected by:

- **Required behaviour** — e.g. what the situation demands. A dangerous task such as trampolining requires an autocratic approach, to maintain safety.
- **Actual behaviour** — e.g. the style and approach the leader decides to take. This is based on their own ability and other factors. For example, the leader considers all the factors and decides to use an autocratic style of leadership.
- **Preferred behaviour** — e.g. the style of leadership preferred by the performers based on their own characteristics, such as ability. For example, the group members like the autocratic approach because they develop their basic skills and can move on to more difficult skills quickly.

The leader must try to balance the style of leadership with each of these factors to gain the highest level of performance and satisfaction from the group. The more the leader's actual behaviour matches what the group wants and what the situation requires, the better the performance will be. In the trampolining examples mentioned above, the leader decides to use the autocratic style, which matches what the group likes and what the situation requires, so there is a good chance that performance will improve and the group will be satisfied.

> **Tip** Many students find Chelladurai's model difficult. Try working backwards through the model to explain it, describing each box in your answer and what it means. Always give clear examples and when working through a model, use the same example throughout.

Evaluating contemporary influences in sport

Concepts and characteristics of World Games

What the examiner will expect you to be able to do

- Identify key characteristics of World Games and their impact on the individual, the country and the government.
- Identify the stages of Sport England's development continuum and explain various socio-cultural factors influencing progression through it.
- Explain the role and structure of the world-class performance pathway.
- Identify and explain how various organisations are supporting the progression of performers through to elite level.

Key characteristics of World Games

Global sporting events (i.e. World Games) can be identified by a number of key features:

- they attract the best elite performers to decide the world's number one positions
- there is a high level of commercialisation linked to world-wide media coverage
- they may be multi-sport (e.g. the Olympics) or single-sport (e.g. the football World Cup)
- they bring nations together in a sporting festival atmosphere (i.e. integration)
- they promote nation-building — for example, developing national pride by showing a country in its best light through hosting or being successful in the Olympics, as in China and Beijing in 2008
- there may be deviancy (e.g. drug use or cheating)

Impact of World Games

For a **host nation and government** elite global sporting events are important for a number of reasons. For example, they:

- increase the status and aid promotion of a host city and country internationally (e.g. London 2012)
- promote social inclusion, improve cultural relationships and integration
- lead to regeneration and improvements to infrastructure such as transport links and leave a positive legacy of sports facilities, athlete accommodation blocks etc.
- encourage success among national performers through heightened national pride in hosting a world event
- bring economic benefits through tourism and employment opportunities
- encourage participation and health and fitness through positive role models

Hosting global sports events also has potential benefits for **individuals**:

- the opportunity to represent their country on home soil
- the opportunity to perform at the highest level and seek recognition as the best in the world — pride in their achievement, fame and extrinsic rewards may result
- the opportunity to develop friendships in a spirit of 'friendly sporting rivalry' (i.e. cultural integration)

Critics argue that there are also a number of potential **drawbacks** for hosts. Businesses and homeowners may be forced to relocate to accommodate infrastructure developments. There may be overcrowding and disruption to everyday life. Debts and/or high costs to the taxpayer may be incurred if the games are not commercially successful. There may be an increased threat of terrorism. Finally, there may be a legacy of unused facilities after the games if this is not thought through at the planning stage.

Sport England's sport development continuum

The **participation pyramid** illustrates the progressive development of an athlete from beginner (foundation) to elite (excellence) level.

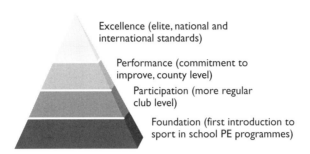

Excellence (elite, national and international standards)

Performance (commitment to improve, county level)

Participation (more regular club level)

Foundation (first introduction to sport in school PE programmes)

Factors influencing the progression to sports excellence

The **physical and psychological qualities** necessary to become an elite performer include:

- high level of ability and natural talent
- high level of skill and fitness
- correct somatotype (body type)
- motivation and long-term commitment to train; determination to be the best
- control of arousal levels
- ability to accept constructive feedback
- mental toughness, readiness for self-sacrifice, high level of self-confidence

The **social and cultural influences** that can affect a child's participation in a particular sport and therefore possible progression include:

- tradition of sports participation
- popularity of sport at school
- positive role models and/or media coverage to inspire participation
- structured levels of competition
- parental influence or pressure, family support and religious preferences
- teacher's speciality and interests
- accessible facilities for different activities near home
- availability of specialist coaching, sports science support etc.

Talent identification and development programmes

Working in partnership, UK Sport, the English Institute of Sport (EIS) and national governing bodies (NGBs) of sport are committed to systematically unearthing sporting talent with the necessary potential and mindset to win medals and world titles. Wherever **talent identification** and development programmes take place, they need to consider:

- physiological factors, e.g. fitness
- anthropometry, e.g. height in volleyball and rowing
- psychological factors, e.g. mental toughness
- hereditary factors or natural advantages
- sociological cultural factors, e.g. family support

There is an important link between the participation level and the excellence level on the participation pyramid: the larger the base of participation, the greater the number of athletes who will filter towards the top. Therefore, it is important that the base of talent is widened. One effective method is to centre the search in schools, as this reaches the maximum number of children. In addition, sports themselves need to become more open and democratic by reducing the incidence of racial, sexual and class-based discrimination.

Reasons for using talent identification programmes

- All potential performers can be screened.
- Performers can be directed to sports most suited to their talents.
- The development process can be accelerated.
- Efficient use can be made of available funding.
- The chances of producing medallists are improved.
- They provide a coordinated approach between organisations.

Talent identification programmes have some drawbacks. For instance, they may miss 'late developers'; they are viewed by some as expensive and give no guarantee of success; and they may lead to early specialisation with too much physical stress and psychological pressure to succeed.

What makes a talent identification programme effective?

- Simplicity of administration and record-keeping, and clear division of roles.
- Talent identification monitoring systems that are built on good practice and appropriate tests.
- Provision of sports services (e.g. sports scientists, physiotherapists) to support performers.
- Well-structured competitive programmes and development squads at various levels appropriate to participants' current level of performance.
- Specialist facilities to support progression.
- Funding at different stages of development.
- Performance-lifestyle support to cope with competing demands of sports partici- pation and work, education, family life etc.

Support structures to help elite development

Support provided	By whom?
Financial support and investment, e.g. World Class Pathway (WCP), Athlete Personal Award (APA), Talented Athlete Scholarship Scheme (TASS)	NGBs, family, SportsAid, sponsorship, UK Sport, National Lottery
High-quality coaching and specialist, top- level facilities	EIS, UK Institute of Sport, Sportscoach UK, NGBs, centres of excellence, UK Sport
Sports science (technology, physiotherapy, medicine, nutrition)	EIS, centres of excellence, NGBs, higher education institutions (as part of EIS/TASS funding)
Talent identification	NGBs, UK Sport, EIS regional scouts
Structured, progressive levels of competition and training in elite groups	Academies, specialist schools, sports colleges, county and regional squads, development squads, NGBs, training camps, UK Sport

The World Class Performance programme: funding sports excellence

The UK won 47 medals and finished fourth in the medal table in the 2008 Beijing Olympics. A number of developments have occurred to support UK athletes financially and continue this success. For example, UK Sport has assumed full responsibility for all Olympic and Paralympic performance-related sport in England. UK Sport has announced **World Class Pathways** funding on three levels:

- **podium** — supporting athletes with realistic medal capabilities for the next Olympic/Paralympic Games (i.e. a maximum of 4 years away from the podium)
- **development** — supporting athletes who have demonstrated realistic medal capabilities (typically 6 years away from the podium)
- **talent** — supporting the identification and confirmation of athletes who have the potential to progress to a higher pathway with the help of targeted investment (typically 8 years away from the podium)

Summary of key organisations and sports excellence initiatives	
EIS Excellence institutes throughout the country	• Sports science/sports medicine support • Performance lifestyle support • Top-quality training facilities • Top-quality coaches and elite-level training squads
UK Sport Overall responsibility for development of elite sport in the UK	• Distributes lottery funding for elite performer development • Oversees work of EIS, etc. • World Class Events programme • Promotes ethically fair, drug-free sport
Sport England Assesses NGB Whole Sport Plans for funding	• Responsible for the 'Excel' part of the overall strategy • Works with NGBs to improve talent identification systems in a variety of sports • Finances NGB Whole Sport Plans • Developed Coaching for Young People initiative with the Youth Sport Trust and NGBs
Sports Coach UK 'Great coaches, great sport'	• Attempting to create a world-class coaching strategy • Developing a UK Coaching Certificate to include the development of 'advanced coaches' with a hierarchy to 'master coaches' • Provision of development officers to support the development of elite coaches • 'Coachwise' resources to develop coaches
NGBs Overall responsibility for development of a specific sport, e.g. British cycling	• Identifies and selects performers for WCP, APA and TASS • Appoints performance directors • Trains high-level coaches in their own sports • Developmental training, squads and competitions
British Olympic Association The independent voice for British Olympic sport	• Works with NGBs to select Team GB • Runs British Olympic Medical Institute • Provides an Olympic training centre and preparation camp • Provides Olympic and Paralympic Employment Network (OPEN)

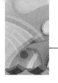

Summary of key organisations and sports excellence initiatives	
National Lottery Major source of funding for elite performer development, supporting performers' quest for global sporting success	• Funds the WCP programme • Provides finance to support warm-weather training, living costs and the APA • Funds top-level training and competition facilities • Funds bids to attract major sporting events to the UK
SportsAid Charitable organisation that receives money from individual donations and fundraising events	• Funds up-and-coming sports performers with a proven financial need • Supported by performers' NGBs • Not in receipt of lottery funding

The 'Olympic ideal' and its place in modern-day sport

What the examiner will expect you to be able to be able to do

- Outline a range of social and cultural factors influencing the development of rational recreation from pre-industrial times to present.
- Explain a number of key influences in the development of rational recreation, such as the Industrial Revolution, urbanisation, the emergence of the middle classes, improved communications, the Church, public provision and the changing nature of working conditions for the masses.
- Explain how rational recreation spread within British society and globally due to the influence of ex-public schoolboys, the formation of NGBs and the emergence of mass spectator sport.
- Compare the historical view of amateurs and professionals in sport with the modern-day view.
- Define the 'contract to compete' and discuss how relevant it is to modern-day elite sport.
- Define what is meant by the concepts of gamesmanship, sportsmanship and the Olympic ideal.

The development of rational recreation

Characteristics of rational recreation

'Rational recreation' involves the post-industrial development of sport. This was characterised by respectability, regularity, stringent administration and codification.

The characteristics of rational recreation are compared with those of 'popular recreation' (physical activity for the masses in agrarian society) in the table:

Rational recreation	Popular recreation
Regular competitions, regionally, nationally, internationally	Occasional events/competitions held locally due to agrarian calendar and limited travel opportunities
Strict codification	Simple, unwritten rules due to illiterate society and lack of structure
Respectable, fair play, non-violent	Violent, unruly, cruel due to harsh nature of society
Control of gambling	Wagering, perhaps a reflection of the society's lack of morals
Purpose-built facilities	Natural/simple environment — what was readily to hand was used
Urban	Rural
Skill-based/tactical	Strength-based/few tactics, reflecting key qualities necessary for survival in the society of the time

Social and cultural influences on rational recreation

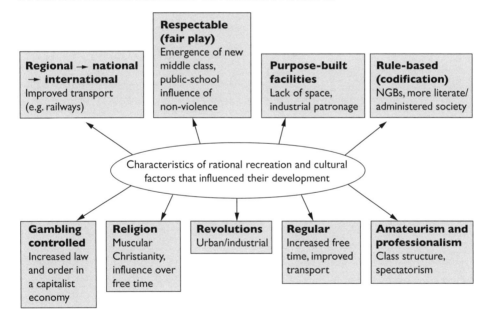

The Industrial Revolution

The influence of the Industrial Revolution on the development of rationalised sports and pastimes changed over the nineteenth century. During the first half of the century, the effects were negative:

- migration of the lower classes into urban areas — loss of space and overcrowding
- lack of time — shift from 'seasonal' to 'machine' time leading to 12-hour days
- lack of income — low wages and poverty

- poor health — poor working and living conditions, lack of hygiene and little energy to play
- loss of rights — restriction placed on mob games and blood sports by changes in criminal laws

In the second half of the nineteenth century, improvements had a positive effect:
- health and hygiene improved
- there was more time for sport due to the factory Acts and Saturday half-day
- development of the new middle class changed ways of behaving and playing sport — it became more acceptable
- influence of ex-public schoolboys via industry, Church etc.
- values of athleticism spread to the lower classes
- industrial **patronage** led to provision for recreation and sport — factory teams, excursions to the seaside etc.
- improvement in transport and communications influenced the distances spectators and players could travel, and leagues were established
- it became cheaper to travel

Urban industrial factors

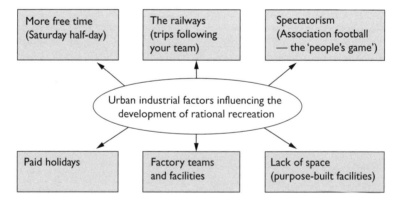

Changes in working conditions as a result of the Industrial Revolution affected participation. **Industrialisation** meant that people often spent 72 hours a week at work in factories, although hours gradually reduced and **holidays** (a single week or day) became regular for all, giving some time for sport. Excursions and workers' sporting facilities provided by some employers also gave opportunities. Free time, however, was very limited — church attendance was expected on Sundays and absenteeism from work was discouraged. **Urbanisation** meant there was a lack of space, which led to a gradual increase in the provision of public parks and swimming baths. This meant that people could gather to watch sport, encouraging **spectatorism**.

The transport revolution
The railways increased participation opportunities and spread interest in sport. Faster trains enabled people to travel further and more easily, giving more time for sports matches. Spectators could follow their teams to away matches and regular fixtures

developed, creating a need for unified rules or **codification**. Field sports, climbing and walking all became more accessible. Although trains were expensive and used mostly by the middle and upper classes, excursions, often sponsored by employers, allowed working people to travel.

The influence of the Church

Changing views of the Church during Victorian times also helped to promote sport and recreation. Sunday-school teams encouraged social control through 'civilised' activities. Church facilities such as halls provided venues for 'improving the morality' of the working classes. The development of the YMCA promoted the healthy body/healthy mind link. The clergy took an active role so as to increase church attendance.

Reasons for the formation of NGBs

During the mid- to late nineteenth century, NGBs began to develop in England for the following reasons:

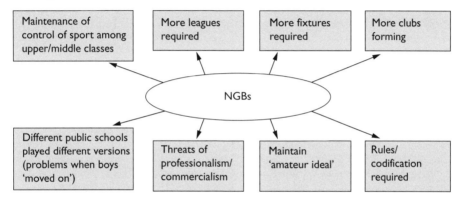

Amateurism and professionalism

Time has changed how **amateurs** and **professionals** are viewed in sports participation. Amateurs are not paid for sporting involvement and tend to play for the love of it. Professionals receive payments for sporting involvement as salaries and winnings, and extrinsic rewards are an important motivator for participation.

The characteristics of a 'gentleman amateur' included:

- being a respected member of society with a public-school background
- belonging to the social elite, having wealth and plenty of free time for sport
- participating in sport as a character-building exercise; training was frowned upon as this would constitute professionalism

The new middle classes admired the cultural values of the upper-class gentleman amateur. They played sport in their free time according to similar principles of amateurism.

The working classes were the poorest members of society and they had to make money from sport or they could not afford to play. The working-class professional came from a poor background and was perceived to be corruptible as he was controlled by money — for instance, he would take a bribe to 'throw' a fight or lose a game on purpose. Early professionals in walking and running races, for example, were paid according to results. Hence training was specialised and winning became the most important thing. The middle and upper classes used the 'amateur code' in most sports to exclude the working classes.

Amateurism (high status in nineteenth century)	Professionalism (low status in nineteenth century)
Came with the onset of the Victorian era (from the mid-nineteenth century)	Slowly developed, with full onset coinciding with the commercialisation and media coverage of sport in the late twentieth century
High morality, sportsmanship and 'gentlemanly' behaviour	Foul play, gamesmanship and cheating to gain an advantage
Games not taken too seriously; winning not important for upper classes	Win at all costs, high rewards at stake and pressure to succeed to maintain lifestyle

Early twentieth-century amateurs	Modern-day amateurs
Held high status in sport and society	Tend to be of lower status (professionals now are of higher status)
Were the best players in their sport	Some high-level performers are still not professional (e.g. gymnasts)
Middle and upper classes controlled sport, excluding (e.g. financially) working classes from amateur sports	Blurring of amateur/professional distinctions, with less likelihood of exclusions as society becomes more egalitarian
More likely that top performers would come from middle or upper classes	Performance at the top level in most sports is now open to all
Had sufficient income/leisure time to play sport for the love of it, receiving no payment	Some amateurs receive finance to pay for training expenses through scholarships or sponsorships

Many factors are responsible for the increased status of professional performers from the early twentieth century to modern day:
- All classes can compete; social class is no longer a barrier to participation.
- People are respected for their talents and efforts in reaching the top.
- There are high rewards for professionals through media and sponsorship.
- Professionals have more time to train, leading to higher standards of performance.
- Celebrity status, more media coverage and role models act as motivators to achieve in professional sport.

The contract to compete

In all sporting situations, there is an unwritten contract — a mutual agreement between opponents — to strive 100% to assert themselves over one another within the rules, allowing a fair opportunity to achieve the ultimate objective of winning. It involves acceptance of the need for codes of behaviour (i.e. **sportsmanship**) as opposed to a win-at-all-costs attitude.

In modern elite sport, the Lombardian ethic emphasising a win-at-all-costs attitude is evident as the rewards for success become greater. Sports performers break the rules and the contract as they attempt to win and reap financial rewards. For example, players may dive to win a free kick in football, make a 'spear tackle' in rugby, take drugs to improve performance in athletics, or fix a tennis match to gain financially.

As a nation we encourage respect for the rules and opponents and this is developed in school PE programmes. Some sports have introduced fair-play charters and campaigns to encourage positive ethics, such as the FA's Respect campaign.

The Olympic ideal

The Olympic ideal (from de Coubertin) is a concept that values 'balance in mind and body', with individuals striving to do their best but maintaining respect for ethical principles. The Olympic ideal was fundamental to the modern Olympic Games when they began in 1896. The statement 'The most important thing in the Olympic Games is not to win but to take part' appears on the scoreboard at every Olympics. The Olympic ideal therefore involves:

- an emphasis on participation
- respect for fellow competitors and tolerance of other nations
- winning as a result of one's own efforts
- sportsmanship (i.e. positive qualities in sport; conforming to the rules and etiquette)

Sportsmanship

Part of the amateur and Olympic ideal involves a spirit of fair play and competing within the written and unwritten rules of a sport. Certain sports have a reputation for sportsmanship and high levels of etiquette — for example, in golf conceding a short putt in match play to an opponent. Sportsmanship can be encouraged through:

- fair-play charters and campaigns (e.g. the FA's Respect)
- use of positive role models (e.g. 100% ME and ethically fair, drug-free sport)
- use of technology to improve officials' decision making
- harsher punishment for negative actions in sport

Gamesmanship

This involves playing a sport and attempting to gain advantage by stretching the rules to their limit, for instance time-wasting in football.

Sport, deviance and the law

What the examiner will expect you to be able to do

- Explain the positive and negative forms of deviance in relation to players, performers and spectators, with examples.
- Identify causes of violence in sport in relation to the player, performer and spectator, and discuss the implications of violence in sport for the player, performer, spectator and the sport.
- Identify and explain possible strategies for preventing performer and spectator violence.
- Give reasons why elite performers may use illegal drugs to aid performance and discuss the implications this has for the performer and the sport.
- Outline different ways in which drug-taking can be discouraged and eliminated, and explain arguments for and against drug-taking and -testing.
- Identify how the law relating to sport is increasingly relevant to performers, officials and spectators.

Deviancy is behaviour that goes against the norms of society.

Positive deviancy is over-adherence to the normal values of society — for example, over-training or performing when injured.

Negative deviancy — the motivation to win at all costs encourages performers who lack moral restraint to act against the norms of society — for instance, taking illegal drugs, deliberately harming an opponent or accepting a bribe to lose.

Violence in sport

Player violence: causes and prevention

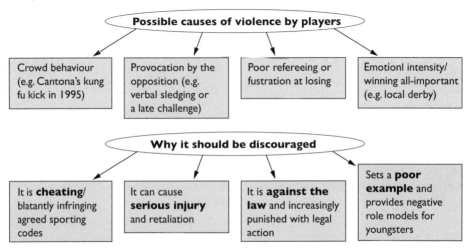

Possible causes of violence by players

| Crowd behaviour (e.g. Cantona's kung fu kick in 1995) | Provocation by the opposition (e.g. verbal sledging or a late challenge) | Poor refereeing or fustration at losing | Emotionl intensity/ winning all-important (e.g. local derby) |

Why it should be discouraged

| It is **cheating**/ blatantly infringing agreed sporting codes | It can cause **serious injury** and retaliation | It is **against the law** and increasingly punished with legal action | Sets a **poor example** and provides negative role models for youngsters |

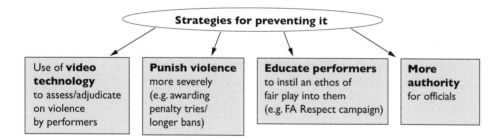

Spectator violence: causes and solutions

Football hooliganism is multi-causal — there are many reasons for it:

- ritual importance of the event, e.g. a local derby
- too much alcohol
- pre-match media hype
- poor crowd control
- diminished responsibility by individuals in a large group (i.e. a football crowd)
- poor officiating
- violence by players on the pitch reflected in the crowd
- religious discord, e.g. at a Celtic versus Rangers match
- taunts by rival fans
- one's own team is losing

Possible solutions include:

- ban on or control of alcohol sales
- use of police intelligence and improved liaison between forces across the country
- tougher deterrents, bans from matches, fines and imprisonment for offenders
- CCTV around stadiums
- removal of terraces, building of all-seater stadiums and segregation of fans
- promoting football as family entertainment and encouraging responsible media reporting

The following table gives some general theories on football hooliganism and comments on how true they are.

General theories	Validity
Young working-class males releasing aggression, thrill-seeking, fuelled by alcohol	Little evidence that working-class males are any more or any less aggressive than other males
Nationalism (seeing other countries' fans as an enemy, encouraged by media hype, e.g. Germany versus England)	Not all international spectators/other sports fans behave like this
Reaction by working-class fans to the takeover of football by middle-class spectators	Hooligans come from a wide range of social backgrounds
Lack of punishment by authorities	Stricter punishments are being given by the authorities
Violent on-pitch actions by players and poor officiating provoke off-pitch violence	Some 'violent' sports are not linked to hooliganism (e.g. rugby; fans' passions are under control)

Drug-taking in sport

The desire to win at all costs in the competitive world of modern sport means that performers continue to take drugs illegally despite the obvious risks. The specification requires an understanding of the reasons why sports performers take drugs and ways in which drug-taking can be eliminated.

Why athletes take performance-enhancing drugs

The reasons can be grouped as follows:
- **Physiological reasons** — to build muscle, power and strength (e.g. anabolic steroids); to enable athletes to train harder and increase energy.
- **Social reasons** — extrinsic rewards that come from success, such as money and fame; pressure to win from coaches, peers, the media and sponsors; drugs are easily accessible and there are few deterrents.
- **Psychological reasons** — to steady nerves (e.g. beta blockers); to increase aggression (e.g. anabolic steroids); to increase confidence (e.g. stimulants).

Reasons for banning performance-enhancing drugs

The use of performance-enhancing drugs gives an unfair advantage to the drug-taker and it is against the International Olympic Committee's fair-play ethic. It is also illegal in the case of certain drugs and can have adverse effects on health, such as addiction and heart disorders.

The negative consequences if an athlete is caught include bans, loss of medals, prestige and earnings, and damage to the reputation of the sport — for instance, the 2007 Tour de France became the 'Tour de Farce' owing to the number of competitors testing positive. There is concern about the negative example drug-taking gives to children and the encouragement it may give to other athletes.

Arguments supporting the legalisation of drugs

If properly monitored, performance-enhancing drugs do not present a health risk. Many drugs occur naturally and some are used for normal medical care, so it is difficult to define the line between nutritional substances and illegal drugs. Athletes don't ask to be role models and the time and money spent on testing could be spent elsewhere. In many cases testing has proved ineffective because it has not caught the cheats, and it can be unsound, jeopardising athletes' careers — as happened with Diane Modahl.

Strategies and difficulties in preventing drug-taking

Most people feel the fight to discourage and eliminate drug-taking in sport should continue. Possible strategies include:
- random and out-of-competition testing, and increased investment in testing
- better coordination between organisations (e.g. the World Anti-Doping Agency, UK Sport, NGBs etc.) and unified policies from governing bodies
- campaigns and education programmes for coaches and athletes encouraging ethically fair drug-free sport (e.g. 100% ME) including the use of role models

- stricter punishments, life bans and the removal of lottery funding if an athlete tests positive

The problems in eradicating drugs from sport include the following:
- It is difficult to test successfully due to masking agents, the development of new drugs and the need to keep up with scientific advances.
- Drugs are often taken accidentally — for instance, stimulants are found in some cold cures and nasal sprays, as was the case with Olympic skier Alain Baxter.
- Many nutritional supplements contain banned substances, which are not always apparent on the label.
- Different countries and sports have different regulations — for example, football's resistance to accepting the 'whereabouts' rule.
- Widespread testing and its associated legal work result in resources being devoted to defending cases against sports organisations and governing bodies.
- It is difficult to gain access to athletes during training, particularly at training camps abroad.

Sport and the law

The needs of various groups have to be taken into account.

Performers
Performers are linked to the law in different ways through:
- **employment rights and protection**, contractual issues (e.g. the Bosman ruling on freedom of contract) and sponsorship deals
- **drug-testing**, as performers have the right to appeal against NGB and BOA sanctions
- **match-fixing cases** (e.g. Hansie Cronjé)
- **violence on the field of play and compensation claims** or legal actions (e.g. Joey Barton at Manchester City following a training-ground incident)
- **libel actions** against the media (e.g. David Beckham)
- **equal opportunities legislation** (e.g. disability or race discrimination cases)

Officials
A duty of care exists for officials — there have been prosecutions when this has failed (for example, injury due to a scrum collapsing in rugby union). Allegations of bribery have been made, involving the law.

Spectators
Legislation has been brought in to control the behaviour of fans so they act within the law — for instance, there should be no pitch invasions or racist chanting. Clubs have a responsibility to fans to ensure their health and safety, so there should be all-seater stadiums, ticket controls, no fencing and control of alcohol sales.

Commercialisation in modern-day sport

What the examiner will expect you to be able to do
- Explain the advantages and disadvantages to the performer, coach, official, spectator, sport and World Games of commercialisation, sponsorship, the media and technology.

Sport, the media and business

The 'golden triangle'

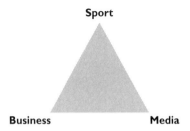

Sport, the media, business and sponsorship are inter-linked and mutually dependent — the 'golden triangle'. For instance, without media coverage, sports are less attractive to sponsors which want their business or product to be publicised to as many people as possible. The media use sport to gain viewers, listeners and readers. In turn, businesses and sponsors use the media to advertise their products and services: organisations often pay substantial sums to sport and the media for advertisements.

Commercialism, media and sponsorship

There is massive media interest in certain high-profile sports — television companies pay huge amounts of money for the right to show a sporting event, e.g. football on Sky Sports — as sport has a positive image. Sponsorship deals result from television exposure. Merchandising too relates to media exposure — clothing and equipment companies such as Nike and Adidas have become strong rivals in sponsoring teams and individuals to aid their merchandising.

Governing bodies and other organisations have become multinational companies. For example, the US National Basketball Association (NBA) and National Football League (NFL) have spread their influence and products around the world in 'demonstration' games.

Agents seeking the best for their clients thus have increasing control over performers.

Characteristics of commercial sport
Commercial sport has close links with:

- **professional sport** — it is high quality
- **sponsorship and business** — they go hand-in-hand
- **entertainment** — watching sport is part of a mass-entertainment industry
- **contracts** — e.g. involving sales of merchandise and television rights
- **athletes as commodities** — e.g. as an asset to companies through product endorsement, which brings increased sales
- **wide media coverage** — and interest in high-profile sports that are visually appealing and have high skill levels, well-matched competition and simple rules

Advantages and disadvantages of commercialisation

Advantages	Disadvantages
• Provides money for sport, leading to improved resources, facilities and coaching	• Success becomes the main focus, encouraging deviant behaviour, cheating and gamesmanship
• Leads to more events (e.g. growth of Twenty/20, 50-over cricket competitions)	• Tends to support already popular sports and so the gap with other more 'minority' sports widens (so increasing funding inequalities between sports)
• Provides positive role models and increases a sport's profile, prompting increased participation in sport	• Favours male-dominated over female-dominated, elite over grass-roots and able-bodied over disabled sports, causing further inequalities
• Allows athletes to earn and work full time, so they can train for longer and compete internationally	

Effects of commercialisation on professional performers

As a result of commercialisation, professional sportsmen and sportswomen:

- receive high incomes for sports participation and commercial activities promoting products, which gives financial security and allows full-time training and competition
- are paid for successful results, which makes winning important
- can be put under pressure to perform when injured
- must specialise in a sport in order to compete, which requires serious training, dedication and self-sacrifice
- are effectively entertainers who become household names, e.g. David Beckham, Tiger Woods and Ronaldo
- are controlled by the sponsor, become public commodities and suffer from a lack of privacy

Effects of commercialisation on sport

Some sports have changed as a result of commercial and media interest, for instance:

- rules and scoring systems have been changed or introduced to speed up the action and prevent spectator boredom — e.g. the multi-ball system at football matches cuts down on time-wasting; badminton scores on every point

- breaks are provided in play so that sponsors can advertise their products and services
- competition formats have changed — e.g. Twenty/20 cricket is a major revenue-earner due to spectator, television and commercial interests
- sports played by women receive less coverage, which can affect participation and funding negatively — there are fewer role models and there is less money to reinvest into sport at grass-roots and professional levels
- the increased use of technology through the media has led to a more personal experience for the viewer (e.g. the stump cam in cricket)

Advantages and disadvantages of media coverage

Advantages	Disadvantages
Raises the profile of a sport (e.g. football has a very high profile)	Lowers a sport's profile if there is little or no coverage (e.g. gymnastics)
Raises participation levels (e.g. tennis during Wimbledon fortnight)	Lowers participation if there are no role models to aspire to
More money is available for players, facilities and training opportunities as a result of revenue from television companies in particular	There is a lack of funding for players, facilities and training (e.g. if there is no funding from television companies, a sport is less attractive to sponsors)

Effects of media coverage on the performer

Performers may become concerned with image and the need to sell themselves to attract sponsorship. In response to media pressure, especially tabloid, they may entertain to maintain sponsorship. Acting at all times in a way that fits their celebrity status becomes important; if they fail to do so it is widely reported.

Effects of media coverage on sports competitions

A number of changes to the format of sports contests have been made to accommodate the media. For example, 5 points for a try in rugby was introduced to make matches more exciting. There has been a concentration on more 'entertaining' events to the detriment of others — for example, there is concern that Twenty/20 cricket will overshadow other forms of the game including 5-day test matches. Timings have also been altered to suit television programming — for example, to meet Sky's requirements, Premiership football is often spread from Saturday to Monday evening, rather than being on the traditional Saturday afternoon.

Role of the media in promoting sport in the UK

The media raise the profile of sport by highlighting major competitions and incidents, and turn some sports performers into role models. Wider coverage has increased revenue for some sports (e.g. rugby and football). It has also created commercial opportunities for sports merchandise, as customers want to wear the same kit as their heroes.

Sport has also become more globalised. American football is now well known in the UK, through coverage by Channel 4 then Sky, and it has been promoted by NFL games at Wembley.

Technology in sport

1 Do modern television and related broadcasting technologies give the same spectator experience as attending a live sport event?

Yes — arguments for:
- Enhanced sound and picture quality improves the experience, e.g. high-quality, high-definition digital technology.
- Technology allows individualised experiences through live screenings, player cam, HawkEye and referee link in rugby.

No — arguments against:
- The audience does not get an all-encompassing view and the experience lacks the 'real' atmosphere.
- There is less sense of being part of the spectacle or playing a role in the contest.
- The audience is unlikely to interact with opposition spectators.

2 Are LZR Racer-type swimsuits a help or a hindrance?

	Positives	**Negatives**
Performer	Able to improve performance standards and set more world records	Unfair advantage to performers who wear the suits as they are not available to all Is technology, not training, responsible for improved performances?
World Games	Spectators want to see the highest possible performance standards at global games	Some scepticism about ethics and fairness of the competition
Media and sponsorship	Companies increase investment to gain an edge over their commercial rivals Record-breaking raises profile of swimming in media	Certain companies which feel they are unable to compete with the Speedo LZR Racer may withdraw investment from swimming (e.g. Adidas and Nike)

Questions
&
Answers

This section of the guide contains questions that are similar in style to those you can expect to see in the Unit 3 exam. The questions cover all the areas of the specification identified in the Content Guidance section. One example is given of the type of extended answer required for the 14-mark compulsory question (see Question 11). In the exam you are required to answer a similar 14-mark compulsory question for each of the three topics you have studied (applied physiology, psychological aspects and contemporary influences). The shorter answers given here are typical of those that contribute to the 7-mark questions.

Each question is followed by an average or poor response (Candidate A) and an A-grade response (Candidate B).

You should try to answer these questions yourself, so that you can compare your answers with the candidates' responses. In this way you should be able to identify your strengths and weaknesses in both subject knowledge and exam technique.

All candidate responses are followed by examiner comments. These are preceded by the icon 🖉 and indicate where credit is due. In the weaker answers they also point out areas for improvement, specific problems and common errors, such as vagueness, irrelevance and misinterpretation of the question.

Question 1

Energy sources and systems

(a) **What are the main energy sources used by an athlete during a 400 m sprint? Explain the predominant energy system used during this time.** (7 marks)

(b) **In team games, players need to manage the physiological demands during performance. The diagram below shows the average proportions of carbohydrate and fat used during a period of exercise of increasing intensity.**

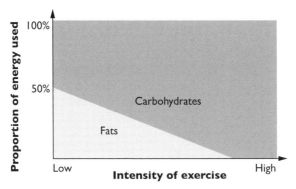

Describe what this diagram shows and explain, using your knowledge of energy systems, why this occurs. (6 marks)

Total: 13 marks

Candidates' answers to Question 1

Candidate A

(a) The main energy sources used by a 400 m runner are carbohydrate ✓ and phosphocreatine ✓. The ATP/PC system is used for the first part of the race and is a simple system to use. It uses phosphocreatine as the fuel and there are no fatiguing by-products. The energy yield is 1 ATP. After 10 seconds the lactic acid system is used.

   Candidate A scores 2 marks out of 7. The candidate has correctly named two energy sources used during the 400 m. The question then asks for the *predominant* energy system, so naming both the ATP/PC system and the lactic acid system is incorrect and scores no marks. The predominant energy system during the 400 m is the lactic acid system and this should be explained.

Candidate B

(a) The energy sources used by the sprinter are phosphocreatine ✓ and glucose ✓. The main energy system is the lactic acid system ✓. This is anaerobic ✓ and glucose is broken down into pyruvic acid ✓. Two molecules of ATP ✓ are formed and lactic acid is the by-product ✓. This system takes place in the sarcoplasm ✓.

> 📝 Candidate B scores the full 7 marks. The correct energy sources are identified and the correct energy system is explained. This answer gives more credit-worthy points than there are marks available.

Candidate A

(b) At low-intensity exercise 50% of energy comes from fats and 50% from carbo-hydrates ✓. This is because fats need more oxygen for their breakdown ✓ so they cannot be used anaerobically ✓.

> 📝 Candidate A scores 3 marks. There were 3 marks available for explaining the diagram but this answer concentrates on the use of fats and misses out carbo-hydrates. Remember, if there is a diagram and you are asked to comment on it, marks will be available for saying what the diagram shows. State the obvious and discuss everything you see.

Candidate B

(b) At low-intensity exercise 50% of energy comes from fats and 50% from carbo-hydrates ✓. As the intensity increases, less fat is used and more carbohydrate is used ✓. At high intensity, carbohydrates are the only energy source ✓. At low intensity, fat and carbohydrates are broken down using oxygen ✓. Fats require more oxygen for their breakdown ✓. They are broken down in Krebs cycle ✓. No fats can be used anaerobically ✓.

> 📝 Candidate B scores the full 6 marks. This answer offers more credit-worthy points than the maximum marks available. Describing what the diagram shows scores 3 marks and then describing correctly the conditions and where fats and carbohydrates are broken down earns a further 3 marks. Marks were also avail-able for mentioning glycolysis and lactate formation.

■ ■ ■

Question 2

Causes of fatigue and the recovery process

(a) At the end of a team game, players may experience EPOC. Define EPOC, give the functions of the fast and slow components of EPOC and explain how these functions are achieved. *(7 marks)*

(b) Temperature regulation can be a problem during exercise, especially when the activity is very demanding. Why does an increase in body temperature cause problems and how could a marathon runner regulate his temperature during a race? (7 marks)

Total: 14 marks

Candidates' answers to Question 2

Candidate A

(a) EPOC stands for excess post-exercise oxygen consumption ✓. The fast component involves replenishing ATP and PC stores ✓ and myoglobin levels ✓. The slow component involves getting rid of lactic acid ✓.

🖉 Candidate A scores 4 marks. The candidate has correctly explained EPOC and the functions of the fast and slow components but has not answered the last part of the question. Missing out parts of questions is a common failing in exams, so make sure you check your work.

Candidate B

(a) EPOC = excess post-exercise oxygen consumption ✓. The fast component involves the restoration of ATP and PC ✓ and the resaturation of myoglobin with oxygen ✓. The slow component is the removal of lactic acid ✓. It is possible to get rid of lactic acid by taking in extra oxygen ✓ and oxidising it to carbon dioxide and water ✓. Some lactic acid can be converted to glycogen ✓ and protein ✓ or it can be sweated or urinated out ✓.

🖉 Candidate B scores 7 marks out of 7 and makes more credit-worthy points than the maximum marks available. The candidate has correctly identified all of the question requirements and answered each part comprehensively.

Candidate A

(b) When a muscle contracts there is heat ✓ and this raises the temperature of the body ✓. If the performer gets too hot he will feel uncomfortable so to cool down sweating occurs ✓.

🖉 Candidate A scores 3 marks out of 7. He/she has explained briefly how an increase in temperature occurs but there is little evidence of how temperature is regulated. This answer is too brief and lacks the understanding that would have been evident if the candidate had revised this section of the specification more thoroughly.

Candidate B

(b) Muscle contractions produce heat ✓. This raises core body temperature ✓. As a result blood viscosity increases ✓ and metabolic processes slow down ✓. Sweating becomes less efficient ✓ and dehydration occurs ✓. Temperature is regulated by the medulla ✓, which causes the blood vessels to vasodilate ✓ and heat is lost through sweating, ✓ radiation ✓ and convection ✓.

🖉 Candidate B scores full marks and this answer gives far more points than the maximum available marks. Questions on temperature regulation usually ask two things: what happens when there is an increase in body temperature and how is temperature controlled? There is more emphasis on temperature regulation in the new specification so make sure you understand it.

■ ■ ■

Question 3

What makes a successful endurance performance?

List five *structural* and/or *physiological* reasons why the VO_2 max of an elite athlete may be greater than that of a fun runner. (5 marks)

Candidates' answers to Question 3

Candidate A

Elite athletes have a greater VO_2 max because they have an increased stroke volume ✓ due to a bigger and stronger heart. They have more red blood cells ✓ and therefore more haemoglobin. They also have more capillaries ✓.

> Candidate A scores 3 marks. The candidate has correctly identified that the question asks for five reasons. This is important because if a question states a number, the examiner will only mark that number and any subsequent answers will not be allocated marks. Unfortunately for Candidate A, stroke volume and hypertrophy of the heart were allocated the same mark in the mark scheme, as were increases in haemoglobin levels and red blood cells. Make sure you cover different areas to ensure each point you make is allocated a mark.

Candidate B

Elite athletes have a greater VO_2 max because they have an increased stroke volume ✓. They also have increased numbers of red blood cells ✓ and mitochondria ✓. OBLA levels are higher ✓ and glycogen and triglyceride stores are increased ✓.

> Candidate B scores the full 5 marks. Five different areas are mentioned to ensure there is no repetition. Marks would have been awarded for mentioning increased A-VO_2 diff, reduced body fat and slow twitch hypertrophy. Questions on this topic usually ask for differences in fitness measures either between males and females or between trained and untrained performers.

■ ■ ■

Question 4

Structure and function of muscles

Describe the sliding filament theory of muscle contraction. (7 marks)

Candidates' answers to Question 4

Candidate A

In the sliding filament theory, a sarcomere contains actin and myosin ✓, which slide over one another and join up. They need energy to do this. Calcium also needs to be released ✓ into the muscle cell to enable a contraction to take place as it neutralises other things in the cell.

> 🖉 Candidate A scores 2 marks. This answer does not contain enough detail and although the candidate has a vague understanding of the theory, the answer needs to give more information using correct technical terms.

Candidate B

Each sarcomere contains actin and myosin ✓. These slide across one another and connect or make crossbridges ✓. ATP is needed to form a crossbridge ✓. Troponin and tropomyosin cover the binding sites of the actin ✓. Calcium is released from the sarcoplasmic reticulum and attracts the troponin ✓, which neutralises the tropomyosin ✓ and releases the binding sites on the actin, allowing crossbridges to occur ✓. Crossbridges constantly attach, detach then reattach ✓.

> 🖉 Candidate B scores full marks. Marks were also available for mentioning H zones, I bands and A bands. This is a new topic area on the specification so make sure you revise it thoroughly.

■ ■ ■

Question 5

Sports supplements and ergogenic aids

Name two illegal ergogenic aids that may be of benefit to an endurance performer, explain how they can help performance, and highlight any possible side effects. (6 marks)

Candidates' answers to Question 5

Candidate A

HGH ✓ is an artificially produced hormone that is used to increase muscle mass ✓. Prolonged use can lead to heart and nerve disease ✓. Steroids also produce muscle growth but can lead to acne and liver or heart disease.

> Candidate A scores 3 marks out of 6. The question asks for two illegal aids that would be useful to an endurance performer. Steroids are illegal but they are used mainly by power athletes. This means that the candidate has lost 3 marks by writing about the wrong aid. The specification states that you should be aware of which type of performer uses which types of aid, so always check the question to see what you need to write about.

Candidate B

HGH ✓ is used by some endurance athletes to increase muscle mass ✓ and decrease body fat ✓. HGH can cause heart and nerve disease ✓, glucose intolerance and a high level of blood fats ✓. EPO ✓ is also sometimes used. It is a hormone that can be artificially made to increase the oxygen-carrying capacity of the blood ✓. It can result in blood clotting and strokes ✓.

> Candidate B scores the full 6 marks. He/she has correctly chosen two aids relevant to an endurance performer, explained what they are and how they help performance, and highlighted their side-effects.

■ ■ ■

Question 6

Specialised training

Elite athletes spend considerable time developing their fitness, using a variety of methods, in order to produce peak performance. Explain why some athletes, such as marathon runners, may choose to spend time training at altitude, and highlight the potential problems associated with altitude training. (7 marks)

Candidates' answers to Question 6

Candidate A

Altitude training can improve the stamina of a performer ✓ because it increases the number of red blood cells the performer has ✓. The problems are altitude sickness ✓ and it is very expensive.

> Candidate A scores 3 marks. He/she does not explain how an increased number of red blood cells helps the performer and has highlighted only one problem associated with altitude training. Look at the mark allocation for each question and this will help you to decide how many points to make.

Candidate B

Altitude training increases the endurance levels ✓ of a performer. This happens because red blood cells increase in number ✓, which enhances the oxygen-carrying capacity of the blood ✓. However, altitude training has disadvantages. On arrival at altitude the partial pressure of oxygen is low ✓, which means that training is very hard ✓ and a loss of fitness occurs ✓. Altitude sickness ✓ may also be a problem.

🖉 Candidate B scores 7 marks. Marks were also available for mentioning erythro-poietin. Questions on altitude training usually ask for an explanation of the method together with advantages and disadvantages.

■ ■ ■

Question 7
Sports injuries

Elite performers are increasingly using hyperbaric chambers to enhance recovery from injury. Explain what this method involves, giving an example of the type of athlete that may find a hyperbaric chamber useful. Give the physiological reasons behind the use of this aid. (4 marks)

Candidates' answers to Question 7

Candidate A

Hyperbaric chambers reduce the recovery time from an injury ✓. The performer enters a chamber that is full of oxygen and this helps them to recover quicker ✓.

🖉 Candidate A scores 2 marks. The answer does not explain what the extra oxygen does to help recovery. The question asks for three things: to explain the method, to give an example of the type of athlete that uses hyperbaric chambers, and to give the physiological reasons why they are used. This candidate has addressed only the first point. Make sure you answer the whole question.

Candidate B

Hyperbaric chambers reduce the recovery time from injury ✓. Wayne Rooney used one before the World Cup ✓. The chamber is pressurised to increase the amount of oxygen that can be breathed in ✓ so more oxygen can be diffused to the injured area ✓. The dissolved oxygen reduces swelling and repairs cells ✓.

🖉 Candidate B scores 4 marks. The answer is detailed and covers all aspects of the question. In the case of specialised rehabilitation techniques, the specification tells you exactly what you have to know for the exam: identify the physiological reasons for their use; discuss which athletes find them useful; and decide whether the measure is effective.

■ ■ ■

Question 8

Mechanics of movement

(a) Identify the forces that act on a player during a game of football when she is running towards the ball, and describe the effects of forces on the flight of the ball when it is kicked towards a team-mate. (7 marks)

(b) Using Newton's three laws of motion, explain how a high jumper takes off from the ground. (6 marks)

Total: 13 marks

Candidates' answers to Question 8

Candidate A

(a) Gravity ✓ and reaction ✓ are the forces that act on the player and the ball.

> 🖉 Candidate A scores 2 marks out of 7. Although gravity does affect the ball, an explanation of how it does this is also needed to score the mark. This question requires knowledge of the vertical forces of weight, gravity and reaction and the horizontal forces of air resistance and friction. Candidate A has been too vague and has not applied knowledge of the forces to the sporting example in the question.

Candidate B

(a) The forces that act on the player are gravity ✓, friction ✓ and reaction ✓. The force provided by the muscles changes the motion of the ball ✓. Gravity pulls the ball down ✓ and air resistance affects the distance the ball travels through the air ✓.

> 🖉 Candidate B scores 6 marks. The candidate correctly mentions the forces that act on the football player and the flight path of the ball. Mention of the reduction of both the vertical component and the horizontal component would score additional marks.

Candidate A

(b) The first law is the law of inertia and this occurs for the high jumper when he changes his state of motion from the run-up to the jump ✓. The second law is acceleration and for the high jumper the more force that is applied, the higher he will jump ✓. The third law is reaction. The high jumper gets the reaction force from the ground ✓.

> 🖉 Candidate A scores 3 marks out of 6. This question requires a definition of each law and the application of each law to the high jump. Candidate A has applied each law but not given a definition, and therefore loses 3 marks. If you are not sure whether the question is asking you to identify each law or define it, do both.

questions & answers

Candidate B

(b) The first law is the law of inertia where the body remains in a constant state of motion unless acted upon by a force ✓. The high jumper changes her state of motion from the run-up to the take-off ✓. The second law is the law of acceleration, where the magnitude of force governs the acceleration at take-off ✓. The direction of force also governs direction of acceleration ✓. The more force that is applied, the more height is achieved ✓. The third law is the law of reaction, where for every force there is an equal and opposite reaction force ✓. The reaction force is a ground reaction force ✓.

🖉 Candidate B scores the full 6 marks. He/she has correctly identified, defined and applied each of the three laws. Marks were also available for mentioning that the ground reaction force needs to generate a large vertical component for high jumping, and for naming a muscle group that is used during the jump, such as the quadriceps.

■ ■ ■

Question 9

Arousal

Explain how an athlete may be affected when performing in front of an audience. (7 marks)

Candidates' answers to Question 9

Candidate A

When performing in front of a crowd a performer reverts to her dominant response ✓. This is the skill she uses when under pressure caused by being observed, e.g. a forehand ground stroke in tennis. This is due to increasing arousal ✓. If the performer is an extrovert she will cope with high arousal because her natural levels of adrenaline detected by the RAS will be low ✓ and she needs to get excited to perform at her best. An introvert is the opposite.

🖉 Candidate A scores 3 marks. This answer starts off well, showing good knowledge, understanding and correct use of technical terminology. However, the candidate does not make enough points to gain full marks. Always make more points than the number of marks available (unless the number of points required is identified). If you give six points for a 5-mark question and one point is incorrect you still gain full marks. This answer finishes disappointingly. You must expand your answer fully to gain credit at A2.

Candidate B

When you are being watched, especially if your parents or other significant people ✓ are in the crowd, you may become nervous. This causes your arousal levels to rise ✓.

If you are at cognitive level, your performance will worsen ✓ as you are not used to performing in front of a crowd. This is known as social inhibition ✓. If you are an expert, you are used to performing with a crowd and can handle the pressure so your performance gets better ✓. This is known as social facilitation ✓. This is made even worse when playing away as you don't have the home-field advantage ✓.

🖉 Candidate B has done the bare minimum to score the full 7 marks. The examiner would have to give benefit-of-the-doubt marks. Ideally the candidate should have discussed the dominant response and its effects. The points about significant others and home-field advantage should also have been expanded.

■ ■ ■

Question 10

Confidence

Using Bandura's model and practical examples, explain how self-efficacy can be developed. (7 marks)

Candidates' answers to Question 10

Candidate A
The coach should use verbal persuasion ✓ to tell the performers that they can do the skill. The coach should control the performers' emotions ✓ and keep them calm when performing the skill. The coach should also remind the performers that they have done the skill many times before and so they can do it again ✓, and get one of their team-mates to demonstrate the skill.

🖉 Candidate A scores 3 marks out of 7. He/she has made the common mistake of thinking that writing 'the skill' is good enough as a practical example. It is not! You must name a skill (e.g. a football penalty). The theory is correct but can only gain 3 marks, which for this question is the maximum that can be awarded to answers without examples — in some cases, no examples means no marks. Give an example with every point you make to ensure you access all the marks.

Candidate B
Bandura suggested that in order to develop self-efficacy the coach should remind the performer of previous accomplishments ✓. For example, if a young diver is scared of diving from the 3m board, the coach could remind him that he successfully jumped off it before and is just altering his body position ✓. The coach could also ask one of the diver's friends to encourage him to dive ✓. This is known as verbal persuasion ✓ and it works best if it is from a significant other. The coach might also ask the friend to dive from the 3m board to show the diver that it can be done ✓. This is known as a vicarious experience ✓ whereby the boy will think, 'Well if he can do it so can I'. Finally, Bandura suggests that the diver should have emotional control ✓. He will be

scared and his coach should teach strategies to calm him down. Once he has experienced these four factors he should be able to complete the dive successfully and his confidence will be boosted.

> 🖉 Candidate B scores 7 marks. This is a comprehensive and well-structured answer. The candidate has addressed all four parts of Bandura's model and has applied it to the same example. This helps to demonstrate the candidate's clear understanding and allows the examiner to award marks with ease.

■ ■ ■

Question 11

Attribution theory

Explain the term 'learned helplessness' using examples from sport. What factors may contribute to a performer experiencing learned helplessness? As a coach, what strategies can you put in place so that performers may avoid it?

(14 marks)

Candidates' answers to Question 11

Candidate A

Learned helplessness is like being a NAF ✓ performer. You don't like performing because you know you will lose ✓. For example, if you played a good team before and lost, you think that you will fail when you play them again ✓. To stop this from happening the coach should:

- give positive feedback to the performer ✓
- develop the performer's self-confidence ✓
- attribute success to him/her ✓ rather than to others

This could be for one sport ✓ such as football or all sports ✓. This is global ✓ learned helplessness.

> 🖉 This is a weak answer (level 1 standard) with such limited information it suggests that the candidate ran out of time. Make sure that you allocate enough time for each question. While there are some credit-worthy points, there is a lack of technical terminology. The candidate has missed the second part of the question and the example is vague. Bullet points are not a good idea in the extended answer as you are marked on the quality of your writing — use full sentences and write in paragraphs. Finally, Candidate A has not made this answer examiner-friendly. He/she has returned to the first part of the question at the end. Although any correct points will still gain credit, it would have been better to put this information earlier in the answer. Drawing up a quick plan before you start would help to avoid this.

Candidate B

Learned helplessness is when an athlete believes that no matter how hard she tries, she will fail ✓. She might think she will fail in all sports, which is global ✓ learned helplessness, and this often causes young people to show avoidance behaviour ✓ and withdraw from sport completely. Specific ✓ learned helplessness means that the performer thinks she might fail in one sport or skill, for example 'I'm rubbish at tennis' ✓ or 'I know I will miss penalties' ✓. The athlete may have had bad experiences in the past ✓. She may have lost every tennis match she has played or missed every penalty she has taken ✓. So she has low self-confidence ✓ and begins to lose all the motivation ✓ she had ✓. She could begin to show NAF ✓ characteristics and when she fails she attributes it internally ✓ to low ability ✓ — for example, 'I lost the tennis match because I have no agility' ✓. If she is successful, she thinks it is a fluke and that it won't be repeated. She will attribute success externally ✓ to luck ✓.

In order to avoid this, coaches should raise the confidence ✓ of their athletes. They could do this by setting achievable ✓ process goals, such as to improve the forehand technique in tennis ✓. It may be useful to use the SMARTER principle when setting goals ✓. The coach should praise and encourage ✓ the performer for any success. Bandura calls this verbal persuasion ✓, when a performer is told that the coach believes that she can be successful. The coach should also remind the performer of previous success ✓, for example the last match she won and how well she did. This is known as performance accomplishments ✓. Attributional retraining ✓ should also be done. This is when the coach encourages the athlete to attribute failure to external ✓ reasons such as luck ✓ and when she wins the coach should attribute this internally ✓ to high ability ✓ as this will develop the performer's self-belief and she will begin to develop NACH ✓ characteristics.

> 🖉 This is an outstanding answer, which the examiner could award the highest level (level 4). The candidate has addressed all three parts of the question and has given clear examples throughout. Remember, on the extended question the examiner does not count the number of ticks. He/she looks at the whole answer, including the theory, examples and quality of written work. This answer is clear, uses correct technical language and is constructed using paragraphs. It would therefore be at the top of the level (13–14 marks).

■ ■ ■

Question 12

Leadership

Identify *three* qualities of a leader and explain, using examples, how individuals become leaders. (7 marks)

Candidates' answers to Question 12

Candidate A

A leader is motivated ✓ and can motivate others. Leaders are skilful ✓ and can be autocratic, which means they become bossy. Or they may be democratic which means they listen to people.

> Candidate A scores 2 marks out of 7. This limited answer gives three qualities of a leader but gains only two marks for this part of the question. 'Motivated' and 'motivate others' appear in the same point in the mark scheme. The second part of the answer is irrelevant. The candidate has not read the question properly and has described leadership styles. Read the question carefully and underline the key points before you start.

Candidate B

Leaders have charisma ✓, excellent communication ✓ skills and can empathise ✓ with others. They have a goal that they want to achieve. Individuals may be pre-scribed or emergent leaders. Prescribed leaders are selected from outside the team ✓. For example, the ECB selected Andrew Strauss ✓. An emergent leader comes forward from within a team ✓. This might be because he is the best player in the team. For example, the most skilful player in my football team became the leader as we all respected him and listened to his advice ✓.

> Candidate B scores the full 7 marks. This is an excellent answer that addresses both parts of the question successfully. The candidate has given more than three correct qualities of a leader but has reached the maximum marks available for this point. He/she then explains clearly prescribed and emergent leaders and supports the answer with examples.

■ ■ ■

Question 13
Concepts and characteristics of World Games

(a) **In attempting to gain fourth place in the London 2012 Olympic medal table, a number of talent identification initiatives have been put in place, such as Sporting Giants and Girls 4 Gold. Explain the features of successful talent identification programmes.** (4 marks)

(b) **Critics of global sporting events such as the Olympics point to their high costs, negative legacy of facilities and overcrowding as key reasons against hosting them. Outline possible counter-arguments against the three criticisms outlined above.** (3 marks)

Total: 7 marks

Candidates' answers to Question 13

Candidate A

(a) Talent identification programmes aim to find youngsters who might be good at sport. It is important to carry out tests in schools that are sports colleges ✓. In these schools different tests can be carried out to see which children have the skills necessary to be a success in sport.

> ✎ Candidate A scores 1 mark. This answer is too brief and focuses on a single point linking talent identification to sports colleges. Further marks could have been gained by expanding on types of tests such as physiological, psychological and motor skills assessments.

Candidate B

(a) Talent identification programmes need to be well funded ✓ and carried out from an early age. Schools linked to clubs are a good way of searching for talent ✓. At school, children can do fitness tests like the 12-minute run or the Illinois agility run ✓. Once you have found the talent, you need to make sure that top coaches are available to develop performers ✓ as well as different levels of competition so athletes can be tested ✓.

> ✎ Candidate B scores of the full 4 marks. This is an excellent answer — it makes a number of relevant points in a succinct manner, and gives examples to illustrate the point about fitness testing.

Candidate A

(b) Hosting the Olympics, e.g. London in 2012, is great for a host country as it helps improve a nation's status in the world. This is called nation building and means that the money spent is well worth it ✓.

> ✎ Candidate A scores 1 mark for giving the counter-argument that high costs are outweighed by potential political benefits to a host nation. No other point linking to the question is made, so no further marks are possible.

Candidate B

(b) While the Olympics cost a lot of money to stage, there are many economic benefits, such as jobs created to boost the economy ✓. If planned properly, the sporting facilities can be used after the event by elite performers and the local community ✓. Finally, the large number of people coming to such an event is good for the host country as it generates tourism and brings in a lot of money ✓.

> ✎ Candidate B scores 3 marks. Direct links are made to the three potential criticisms outlined in the question. Questions on World Games often require knowledge about the advantages and disadvantages of hosting these events.

■ ■ ■

Question 14

The 'Olympic ideal' and its place in sport today

(a) In the early nineteenth century mob football was played as a 'popular recreation' activity. Explain the social factors that led to mob games such as football developing into their rational form. (4 marks)

(b) The Olympic ideal proposes that the most important thing is not to win but to take part. How does this Olympic ideal conflict with the modern-day sporting arena? (3 marks)

Total: 7 marks

Candidates' answers to Question 14

Candidate A

(a) During the early nineteenth century mob games were violent and had no rules. They were not played often as a lot of time was spent at work. Sports developed into their rational form due to urbanisation and industrialisation.

> Candidate A fails to score. The first two sentences are irrelevant as they describe characteristics of mob football, which is not required by the question. No marks can be awarded for simply stating that urbanisation and industrialisation were influential — the question asks for an explanation of the factors identified.

Candidate B

(a) Association football developed from mob football due to a number of social factors. Urbanisation meant there was a lack of space available to play mob games ✓. The development of railways meant fixtures could be played a lot further away (e.g. regionally) ✓. Middle-class factory owners wanted a disciplined workforce that was fit to work, not injured all the time so the game became less violent ✓. Ex-public schoolboys wrote down rules of play that the working classes could understand once they started to go to school ✓.

> Candidate B scores 4 marks. Four relevant social factors are given and explained to earn maximum marks.

Candidate A

(b) Sport today is about winning, not just taking part. A win-at-all-costs attitude is called the Lombardian ethic, which goes against the Olympic ideal ✓.

> Candidate A scores 1 mark. A variety of relevant points are required to score more marks.

Candidate B

(b) To a certain extent, the Olympic ideal is in conflict with sport today as it is now all about winning ✓ with a lot of money at stake (e.g. sponsorship deals) ✓. Performers may cheat to win by taking drugs ✓. There is still some fair play, however, which links to the Olympic ideal — for example, in sport today opponents shake hands with each other at the end of a contest ✓.

> Candidate B scores 3 marks. This answer illustrates clear knowledge and understanding of the relevance of the Olympic ideal in modern-day sport, and makes more points than there are marks available to earn maximum marks.

■ ■ ■

Question 15

Sport, deviance and the law

(a) Explain using examples what is meant by positive deviancy and negative deviancy. (2 marks)

(b) Violent acts on the field of play sometimes occur in sports such as association football and rugby. Outline various causes and possible solutions to performer violence in sport. (4 marks)

Total: 6 marks

Candidates' answers to Question 15

Candidate A

(a) Deviancy is behaviour against what society expects. Negative deviancy occurs often in sport — it is behaviour against the rules, e.g. taking drugs to improve performance and high tackling an opponent in rugby ✓.

> Candidate A scores 1 mark. The focus in this answer is on negative deviancy, which is explained correctly with appropriate examples.

Candidate B

(a) Positive deviancy is when a sports performer 'over-conforms' to what is expected (e.g. Freddie Flintoff and Paula Radcliffe competing when injured) ✓. Negative deviancy involves poor behaviour against what society expects (e.g. accepting bribes to lose a match as Hansie Cronjé did in cricket) ✓.

> Candidate B scores 2 marks. Both terms are explained clearly with appropriate examples to back them up.

Candidate A

(b) A high tackle in rugby should not be allowed as it can cause serious injury. It may make the opposition look for revenge and gives a poor view of sports like rugby if it happens a lot.

✎ Candidate A fails to score. This answer focuses on the negative effects of performer violence. It is irrelevant to the question and cannot be awarded any marks.

Candidate B

(b) Performer violence such as a punch or a head butt on an opponent can be caused by a number of factors, such as a win-at-all-costs attitude ✓. Such a strong desire to win may be due to the high financial rewards at stake. It may be retaliation after an opponent has hit you ✓ or the result of a poor decision by the referee, which winds you up ✓.

A number of possible solutions are being tried to reduce performer violence. These include the use of video replays in rugby for incidents officials might have missed ✓. NGBs such as the RFL and RFU could give tougher punishments like longer bans from taking part ✓.

✎ Candidate B scores 4 marks. This examiner-friendly answer earns full marks. It answers both parts of the question clearly and expands on the points made with appropriate examples to illustrate excellent knowledge of the topic.

■ ■ ■

Question 16

Commercialisation in modern-day sport

(a) Identify reasons why companies such as Vodafone and Arriva invest in sports such as motor racing and athletics. (3 marks)

(b) Explain why certain sports (e.g. Association football) are attractive to the media. (3 marks)

Total: 6 marks

Candidates' answers to Question 16

Candidate A

(a) Vodafone sponsors cricket and motor racing. Lewis Hamilton wears Vodafone on his racing suit. This means that Vodafone gets a lot of publicity to promote its products like mobile phones ✓.

✎ Candidate A scores 1 mark. One relevant point is made and explained well but a variety of points need to be made to score more marks.

Candidate B

(a) Different companies invest in sport, like Arriva does with athletics and Kelly Holmes. They do so because their company name and products become better known ✓ and therefore they sell more products and make more profit ✓. There are also tax advantages for a company if it sponsors sport ✓.

> Candidate B scores 3 marks. This is a succinct answer that makes three relevant points in three short sentences to gain the 3 marks available.

Candidate A

(b) Football is popular and is shown on television because people like to watch it. It is on nearly every day of the week. It is over in 90 minutes, which fits into people's busy lifestyles ✓. People watch football to see their favourite players like Frank Lampard, who is a positive role model to others with his non-stop effort ✓.

> Candidate A scores 2 marks. The answer starts with some irrelevant information, which may waste valuable time in the exam, but the candidate develops two relevant points sufficiently well to earn 2 marks.

Candidate B

(b) All types of media give wide coverage to football for a number of reasons. It is entertaining with a lot of goal action to cover ✓. It can easily be televised as it is performed in a relatively small space (i.e. a football pitch) ✓. It has many celebrities that the public wants to read about or watch and can easily relate to, such as Beckham ✓. It is a game that is quite easy for most people to understand so they are more likely to watch it ✓.

> Candidate B scores 3 marks. All the points made are credit-worthy. The main points made are expanded on and illustrate understanding of the topic.